ESSENTIALS OF HUMAN GENETICS

Prof Bir Bahadur
Former Head, Department of Genetics,
Shadan Institute of P. G Studies, Osmania University, Hyderabad, and
Former Head and Dean, Kakatiya University, Telangana
birbahadur5april@gmail.com

Dr Vasavi Mohan
Sr. Scientist, Genetics & Molecular Medicine, Vasavi Medical & Research Centre,
Head, Department of Cytogenetics, Apollo Healthcare Ltd.,
Hyderabad, Telangana.
greenpastures@gmail.com

Dr K. Prasanna Latha
Scientist (ICMR), Department of Genetics, Osmania University
Former Head, Shadan Institute of P.G. Studies, Osmania University
Hyderabad, Telangana.
p_komaravalli@yahoo.com

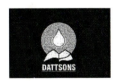

ESSENTIALS OF HUMAN GENETICS

© Author

First Published 2020

ISBN 978-81-7192-191-1

[No part of this publication may be reproduced, stored in a retrieval system or transmitted, in any form or by any means, mechanical, photocopying, recording or otherwise, without prior written permission of the publisher].

Typeset by: PrePSol Enterprises Private Ltd.

Printed at: Anvi Composers, New Delhi

Published in India by
DATTSONS
Jawaharlal Nehru Marg
Sadar, Nagpur-440001 (Maharashtra)
dattsonspublishers@gmail.com

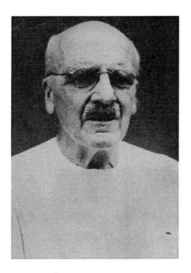

This book is respectfully dedicated to my Mentor, **Prof J.B.S. HALDANE, F.R.S.,** British born Indian, all time great Geneticist and Biologist for inspiration, guidance, and encouragement to the Senior author during 1960-1964.

PREFACE

The pace of advances in genetics will continue to have a lasting impact on our lives for many more decades or even centuries to come, spanning several generations! This no longer remains a question - will genetics shape our future?

This book begins with an introduction highlighting the history of human genetics, followed by mendelian genetics and the DNA era that continues to revolutionize health sciences. The various chapters that follow, aim to provide the reader with information in a phased and coordinated manner. From Gregor Mendel to James Watson to the human genome project, the progress achieved has been beyond expectation. Genetics is the youngest field of biological sciences and has grown vastly during the last 60 years and more, with implications covering many aspects of our life.

The present book 'Essentials of Human Genetics' is intended to introduce the principles of genetics and provide an integrated and utilitarian perspective, wishing to familiarize the science concepts for use by medical and dentistry students alike, as well as for post-graduate and graduate students studying genetics and allied areas. The 30 chapters that follow, cover how genetics has advanced during the last six decades. The book has good reference reading material from basic to molecular, omics, human genome project to so many interesting modern emerging topics, that are relevant to human sciences and research. The book covers topics that overlap both basic human genetics and medical genetics where the study of human genetics answers questions about human inheritance, nature of development, mechanisms that operate to produce various diseases and thus understand their treatment options, ultimately paving the way to understand the future of human life. Medical genetics on the other hand is the branch of medicine that involves the diagnosis and management of various pre-clinical, other medical, hereditary and non-hereditary conditions.

Thanks to the marvellous technological advances, our knowledge of genetics has extended beyond conceivable limits; codes of life have been cracked, tools have been found for probing chromosomes and mysteries of development at the molecular level and so on; thus a wide range of topics has been crisply dealt with, in order to give an over-view, with a simple understanding. The various chapters attempt to reflect basic and applied aspects and presupposes that the reader has familiarity of basic biology and various issues, legal and social. We have gathered information from various sources and sequentially presented it in a lucid way so as to cater to the readers' need to know-how of different topics of current interest. So here's hoping this book makes for good reading

Mastering genetic terminology is critical and crucial to the understanding of the science of genetics. To enable and ensure that the readers grasp and enjoy the subject, an eye-catching self-contained glossary is provided with links to the topics addressed, so that one can delve into areas which stimulate further reading.

We place on record our sincere gratitude to Dr Zeenath Jehan, Senior Scientist, Genetics Unit, Vasavi Medical and Research Centre, Hyderabad for reading the manuscript and for valuable suggestions. We also thank Ms Fatema, Ph.D. scholar, VMRC for her help with figures and proof-reading of the manuscript.

We also wish to express our grateful thanks to our respective family members for their cooperation.

We thank Mr Vinod Nangia, Mr Ankit Nangia and their team of Dattsons Publishers for their professionalism that made this book a reality in a diligent get-up which is greatly appreciated.

We hope that this book will help our readers from different disciplines of biology, teaching, health professionals and researchers who enter the world of the fascinating subject of Genetics with confidence and as we perceived and planned. The readers are requested to give their comments for suggestions for improvement. We also acknowledge that few images used in the book without any reference are in the public domain and generic in nature.

Contents

PREFACE 5

Chapter 1. HISTORICAL BACKGROUND AND INTRODUCTION 11
History of genetic studies, Impact on human disease, Inheritance.

Chapter 2. MENDELIAN GENETICS 17
Mendel's work, Laws of inheritance, History of medical genetics

Chapter 3. CHROMOSOME BASIS OF HEREDITY 35
Theory of inheritance, Mitosis and meiosis divisions and their relevance, Chromosome structures, Genome organization, Molecular organization.

Chapter 4. CYTOGENETICS 44
Banding of human chromosome, Banding techniques, Chromosome nomenclature and abnormalities. Karyotype, Cytogenetic flow-chart, Molecular cytogenetics.

Chapter 5. MOLECULAR GENETICS 54
The central dogma, Watson and Crick model, Classification of DNA, RNA, Genetic code, gene structure, DNA diagnosis, application and DNA banking.

Chapter 6. MUTATIONS...66
History, Kinds of mutations, Physical mutagenesis and genetic effects, Lethal mutations, Autosomal, sex-linked, Qualitative and quantitative, Molecular basis of mutations in humans, Teratogenesis.

Chapter 7. MULTIPLE ALLELES AND POLYGENIC INHERITANCE 76

Chapter 8. PATTERNS OF INHERITANCE 78
Genetic disorders, Single-gene trait inheritance, Autosomal dominant and recessive, Sex-linked and X-linked patterns, Including those of orofacial origin, Y-linked inheritance

Chapter 9. GENETICS OF SYNDROMES 93
Autosomal, Sex chromosomal, Cleft-lip and palate syndromes, Orofacial syndromes

Chapter 10. RARE AND SEVERE GENETIC DISORDERS 102

Chapter 11. DEVELOPMENTAL GENETICS 104
Introduction, Genetic basis, Genes involved in it.

Chapter 12. CANCER GENETICS 108
Cancer biology, Types, Proto-oncogenes, Chromosomal rearrangements and cancer, Tumor suppressor genes, Familial cancer syndromes.

Chapter 13. RADIATION GENETICS 115

Chapter 14. OROFACIAL GENETIC DISORDERS 119
Single gene, Multifactorial disorders, Hapsburg jaw.

Chapter 15. SEX DETERMINATION 123
Sex determination, Chromosomal sex determination system, Sex chromosomes & their abnormalities, Lyonization, Barr bodies, Abnormalities in humans.

Chapter 16. DERMATOGLYPHICS 130

Chapter 17. LINKAGE AND MAPPING 133
Linkage in humans, Human pedigrees, Lod score, gene map, Chromosomal mapping, DNA mapping, Clinical application of linkage.

Chapter 18. MITOCHONDRIAL GENETICS 141
Mitochondrial genome, Inheritance and diseases of mitochondrial origin

Chapter 19. IMMUNOGENETICS 147
Immunogenetics of reproductive biology, Immune response and disease susceptibility

Chapter 20. POPULATION GENETICS 153
Genetic diversity in human populations, Hardy Weinburg equilibrium – salient features, Natural selection, Factors affecting Hardy-Weinburg equilibrium.

Chapter 21. OMICS 158
Genomics, Proteomics, Pharmacogenomics, Other -omics branches - their role in molecular genetics, forward and reverse genetics.

Chapter 22. RECOMBINANT DNA AND GENE CLONING 166

Chapter 23. HUMAN GENOME PROJECT 174
History, Goals, Outcome. Chromosomes with list of genes and important diseases, Internet websites and clinical databases information

Chapter 24. HUMAN BIOMOLECULAR ATLAS PROGRAM 187

Chapter 25. GENETIC COUNSELING 189
Pedigree chart, History, Counselling for orofacial disorders, Mitochondrial diseases

Chapter 26. GENE THERAPY 194
Treatment strategies, Somatic cell therapy, Germline therapy, Social impact, Stem cells

Chapter 27. EUGENICS 200

Chapter 28. CLINICAL GENETIC SERVICES 202

Chapter 29. FORENSIC GENETICS 205

Chapter 30. CRISPR / Cas Technology 208

GLOSSARY 212

Bibliography 219

CHAPTER 1

Historical Background and Introduction

Prior to his death, Mendel wrote, "my scientific work has brought me a great deal of satisfaction and I am convinced that it will be appreciated before long, by the whole world. Sixteen years later in 1900, Mendel's work was re-discovered by three European botanists independently, Hugo de Vries of Holland, Carl Correns of Germany, and Erich von Tschermak of Austria. Within few years of rediscovery, the impact of Mendel's work was felt around the world and was popularly referred as Mendelism. This heralded the birth of the era of Classical genetics. However, it took 40 years before the identification that genetic material is actually Deoxyribonucleic acid, the DNA, thanks to the work of Griffith on *Streptococcus*, followed by Hershey and Chase on T2 phage, and Fraenkel Conrat on Tobacco Mosaic viruses (TMV). Thus, by 1953, the evidence was strongly supportive of nucleic acid as the genetic material to control phenotype, able to replicate, direct protein synthesis and located on the chromosome. Mendel's work remained unappreciated and unnoticed for several decades and unfortunately overlapped with the dawn of the Golden Age of Cytology, when the chromosomes were visualized by Walter Sutton (1903) and Theodore Boveri (1902). Their theory of chromosomal inheritance identified chromosomes as the carriers of genetic material. DNA science was born on 25th April, 1953 when James Watson and Francis Crick published their work on the structure of double helix. This heralded the DNA era which captured the attention of the young and old and the science of Molecular genetics/biology was born (Max Delbruck and Schrodinger). The work on nucleic acid, deciphering of the genetic code, the tools and technologies of genome sequencing, DNA cloning and proteomics have advanced beyond expectations, revolutionized genetics with an exciting challenge of the future to further unravel the intricate and hidden complexity of both, the DNA and RNA.

The first Nobel Prize in Genetics was awarded to Thomas Morgan Hunt in 1933 for his work on chromosome theory of inheritance. This was followed by many others for their discoveries of genetic recombination, the relationship between genes and proteins and the genetic code, genetic regulation of organ development and programmed cell death (Brenner, Horovitz, and Sulston), the role of RNA in gene regulation (Andrew Fire and Craig) and expression, molecular basis of eukaryotic transcription

(R.Kornberg), gene targeting technology essential to the creation of knock-out mice serving as animal model of human disease. The use of various model organisms ranging from phages to bacteria, fungi, lower and higher plants, and various animals used in conjunction with the recombinant DNA technology greatly elucidated various human diseases as briefly summarized below.

Escherchia coli: Colon bacteria- colon cancer and other cancers. Despite the fact that it is a commensal organism, some types contribute to inflammation while toxic gene products from certain other phylogroups together may contribute to cancer risk in the colon. *E.coli* is a key tool in molecular genetics in many genetic manipulations, effectively used in recombinant protein production and molecular cloning is done in one of its vector plasmids in most laboratories.

Saccharomyces cerevisiae: Baker's yeast – cancer risk and Werner syndrome. Yeast was the model organism into which mutations were introduced and biological aspects of gene function was understood. More than a third of S.cerevisiae ORFs (open reading frame) have a mammalian homologue and many genes have been used in modeling human disease; the cellular phenotypes where Sgs1 is disrupted in the organism have reduced life span and the same in humans is associated with a premature aging condition called Werner syndrome.

Drosophila melanogaster: Fruit fly - disorders of the nervous system. Drosophila has complex behavioural patterns including learning and memory making it a system of choice in the study of neurodegeneration.

Caenorhabditis elegans: Round worm – diabetes. Research done on round worms is close to offering a solution to the enigma of a worldwide epidemic like diabetes. Due to its short lifespan, the results of experimental interventions like treatment with metformin and its effects on anti-aging have been described using this organism.

Danio rerio: Zebra fish - cardiovascular diseases. The ability of this organism's heart to regenerate cardiac tissue throughout its lifetime has offered novel approach of understanding regeneration of cardiac tissue in humans. It is a low-cost organism that has been suitably used for forward and reverse genetic studies.

Mus muscularis: Fragile X syndrome, Lesch-Nyhan disease, Cystic fibrosis and other diseases. Mice models have been used in innumerable studies on evolution and conservation, developmental regulation and networks linking genes and disease.

The problems of translating research done on these organisms to humans remain, nevertheless, these studies have provided us with huge amount of information that can be extrapolated to humans, despite skepticism in this regard.

From Mendel's work on inheritance in pea plant in 1965, the molecular basis of gene regulation by Jacob, Lwoff, and Monad (1965) and subsequent spectacular developments that culminated in the completion of Human Genome Project and Human Proteomics Project (ongoing) stand as landmarks for development, advancement and clear indication that we live in the AGE OF GENETICS!

Today, the work on genomics (both structural and functional) focuses on describing the gene expression in various cells in healthy and diseased persons thereby revealing the genetic distinctions that underlie human individuality.

New investigative molecular techniques and new knowledge during the last few decades have greatly helped integration of genetics into biology and medicine. Genetics thus is relevant to practically all medical specialities since the knowledge of basic genetics, principles, and their application in clinical diagnosis are becoming an essential and integral part of medical education and medical practice.

Having a sense of the history of genetics should provide the reader with a useful framework as one proceeds through this book page by page'.

The science of inheritance is called genetics, a term derived from the Greek root "**Gen**", which means to become or to grow into something. It signifies that genetics deals not only with the transmission of hereditary factors but also with the ways in which they express themselves during the development and life of the individual. Inherited variation in the genome is the corner stone of human and medical genetics. Figures 1.1, 1.2 and 1.3 depict the evolution of this advanced science over centuries to what form we visualize it in, as today's most sought after subject that can provide answers to the heritance of human disease and other factors that influence it.

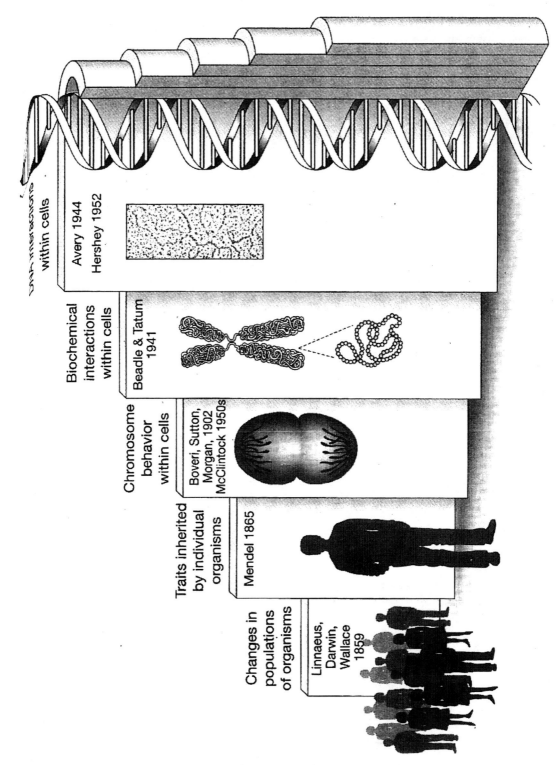

Figure 1.1: Evolution of Science into the era of genetics

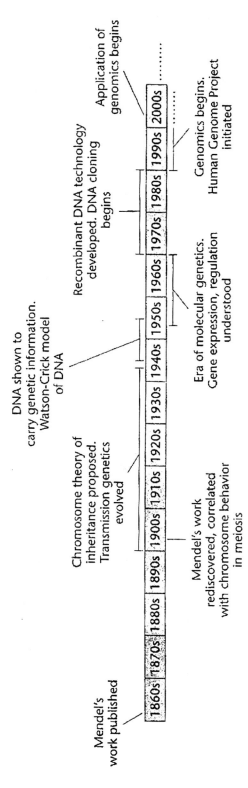

Figure 1.2: A timeline showing the development of genetics from Mendel's work on pea plants to the current era of genomics/proteomics and its many applications in research, medicine & society and agriculture.

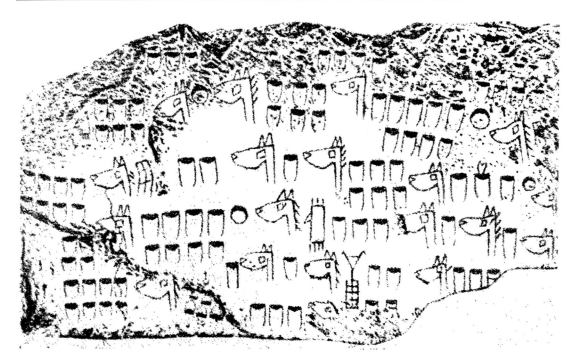

Figure 1.3: Pedigree showing that horse breeding in respect of mane characters was carried out in Chaldea 6000 Years ago (Muntzing, 1961).

2 Mendelian Genetics

CHAPTER

The term Genetics derived from the Greek word meaning to "generate" / "produce" was proposed in 1906 by William Bateson. Genetics is an empirical, young, exciting and evolving science, and deals with the study of inheritance of traits in an organism including human traits in a family pedigree, to biochemistry of the genetic material, the deoxyribonucleic acid. A number of geneticists during its short history of hundred years have researched in various areas, each with its own problems, terminology and organisms. Currently, three broad areas are recognized. *Classical genetics* (transmission genetics) is concerned with the chromosomal theory of inheritance, gene mapping etc, *molecular genetics* deals with the study of genetic material, replication, expression, *r-DNA* (recombinant DNA) technology, genetic engineering including human genome project, while *evolutionary genetics* is the study of evolutionary changes in gene frequencies in populations. Today, these areas are less clearly defined because of rapid advances in molecular genetics and the sophisticated technologies that are associated with it.

(a)
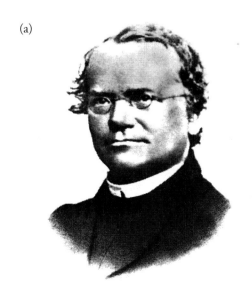

(b)
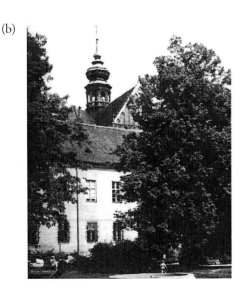

(c)

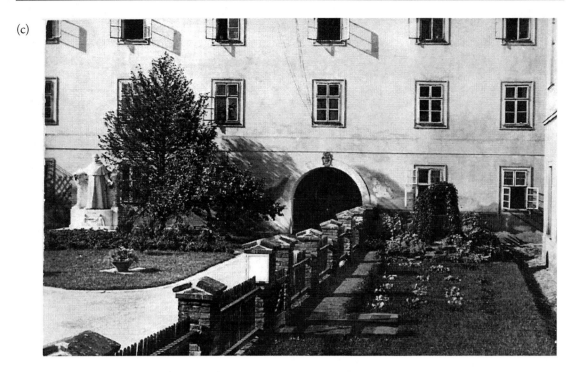

(d)

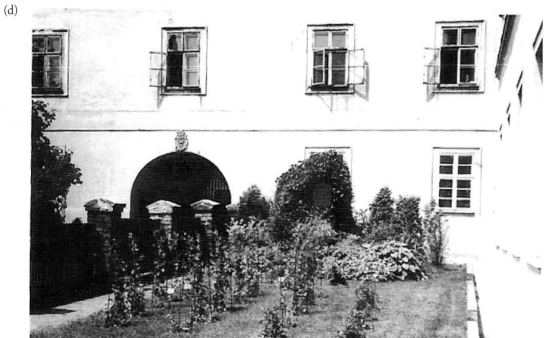

Figure 2.1: (a) 19th century priest, Gregor Mendel (b) Mendel's garden at Brno Augustinian Monastery (c & d) Site of the pea plant experiment (original pictures showing the tall and dwarf pea plants – *Courtesy – Director, Mendel's garden and Museum, Brno*)

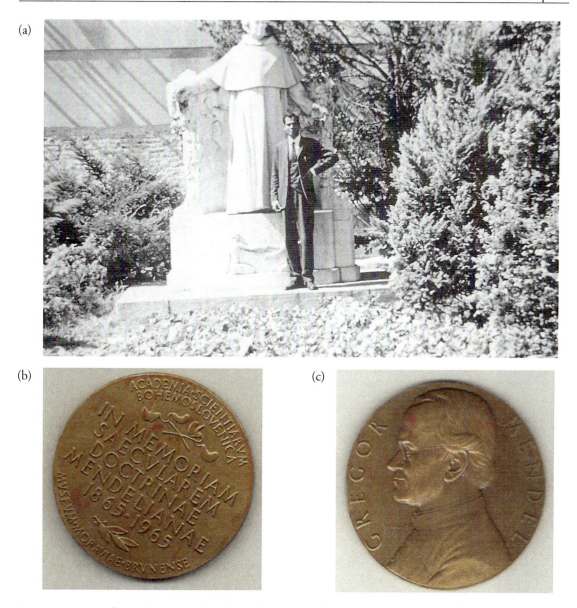

Figure 2.2: (a) Prof Bir Bahadur (Author 1) standing at Mendel's famous garden in 1969 (b & c) Medal released at the time of centenary celebrations (1965) in memory of the famous priest who converted to a scientist.

Our knowledge of genetics has its roots in Mendelian principles or Mendelism. Gregor Johann Mendel (1822-1884) was born in Brunn, Austria on 22nd July, 1822 now in Czech Republic. In 1847, he adopted the name Gregor and was ordained a priest. During 1856–1868, he conducted his famous crossing experiments on garden pea (*Pisum sativum*) an annual plant which grows easily, easy to maintain and easy to cross (Figure 2.1). He selected seven contrasting sets of characters. He crossed two varieties of pea plant considering one pair of contrasting character at a time and obtained hybrids called F_1 generation. Figure 2.2 shows the author in Mendel's garden and the medals in the memory of the famous scientist.

In 1865, Mendel published his findings in a local journal. Unfortunately, this paper remained in obscurity until 1900 when it was rediscovered independently by three botanists - Hugo de Vries in Holland, Erich von Tschermak in Austria and Carl Correns in Germany. Seven characteristics of pea plant in his crossing experiments were observed by Mendel in peas. The traits on the left column are dominant and the alternative forms are recessive.

Alternative forms of alleles/characters

I	Characters of **Seed:**	1) Round	–	Wrinkled
		2) Yellow cotyledons	–	Green cotyledons
		3) Grey seed coat	–	White seed coat
II	Characters of **Pod:**	4) Full	–	Constricted
		5) Green	–	Yellow
III	Characters of **Stem:**	6) Axial pods and flowers along stem	–	Terminal pods and flowers on top of stem
		7) Tall 6'- 7'	–	Dwarf ¾ – 1ft

Genetics can be easily understood if some basic terms are borne in mind. The following terminology is used in describing genetic phenomena. A glossary of terms used in the book is appended to enable the reader to comprehend the subject easily. A few terms are being introduced as a prelude.

1. Mendel's particulate hereditary factors or elements called **genes.** They interact with the environment to determine a particular trait. The term gene was proposed by Danish biologist Wilhelm Johannsen in 1909.
2. The various forms of a given gene are called allelomorph or simply **alleles.**
3. A **locus** is the specific physical region of a gene on the chromosomes.
4. Organisms in which the members of a pair of alleles are different, as in the Aa hybrids are said to be **heterozygous** (generally a carrier in humans), and those in which the two alleles are alike are said to be **homozygous.** An individual organism may be homozygous for the **dominant** (AA) or for the **recessive** (aa) allele, and in both cases will be breeding true for the characteristic determined by the particular allele.
5. The **genotype** is the genetic constitution of an individual. A pea plant contains two alleles of each gene - AA, Aa, and aa are examples of organism genotypes. Because gametes contain only one allele of a given gene, A and a are examples of gamete genotypes. Genotypes are usually designated incompletely in that only the alleles of genes of interest are specified.
6. The observable properties or the sum total of external features of an organism constitute its **phenotype.** Dominance results in the expression of the same phenotypic character - for example,

tall plants - by both the homozygous dominant alleles (AA) and the heterozygous alleles (Aa) genotypes. Johannsen proposed the terms genotype and phenotype.
7. **Autosomal** means autosomes i.e. non-sex chromosomes.
8. **Punnett Square**

The genotypes and phenotypes resulting from the recombination of gametes during fertilization can be easily visualized by figuring a **Punnett's square or Punnett's Check Board,** so named after **Reginald C. Punnett,** the person who first devised this approach. Illustrated here is this method of analysis for the $F_1 \times F_1$ monohybrid cross. All possible gametes are assigned to a column or a row, with the vertical column representing those of the female parent and the horizontal row those of the male parent. After entering the gametes in rows and columns, the new generation is predicted by combining the male and female gametic information for each combination and entering the resulting genotypes in the boxes. This process represents all possible random fertilization events. The genotypes and phenotypes of all potential offspring are ascertained by carefully reading the entries in the boxes (Table 2.A). Subsequently, it was shown that the chromosomes bear genes that were associated with the various characteristics (seven) in the Pea plant, paving way for linkage and mapping studies (Figure 2.3).

The Punnett square method is particularly useful when one is first learning about genetics and how to solve genetic problems. Given below, 3:1 phenotypic ratio and the 1:2:1 genotypic ratio may be derived in the F_2 generation. Figures 2.3 and 2.4 denote the specific characteristics that were studied as part of the experiment and the outcome thereof.

Cross of tall and dwarf pea plants

Parents	Phenotype :	Tall plant	Dwarf plant
Parents	Genotype :	AA ×	aa
Parents	Gametes :	A	a

F_1 progeny : Aa (tall plants)

F_2 progeny : Aa × Aa

Punnett's check Board

Female \ Male	½ A	½ a
½ A	¼ AA	¼ Aa
½ a	¼ Aa	¼ aa

= ¼ AA : ½ Aa : ¼ aa

Table 2.A. Results of Several Characters of Mendel's Experiments

Parental characteristics	F_1	Number of F_2 progeny	F_2 ratio
Round × wrinkled (seeds)	Round	5475 round, 1850 wrinkled	2.96:1
Yellow × Green (cotyledons)	Yellow	6022 yellow, 2001 green	3.01:1
Purple × White (flowers)	Purple	705 purple, 224 white	3.15:1
Inflated × constricted (pods)	Inflated	882 inflated, 299 constricted	2.95:1
Long × short (stems)	Long	787 long, 277 short	2.84:1

(The F in the F_1, F_2 terminology is used for filial, referring to sons or daughters.)

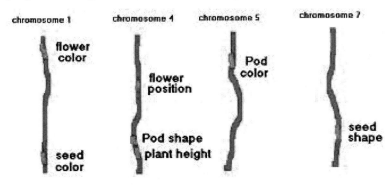

Figure 2.3: Chromosomes with genes for specific characteristics

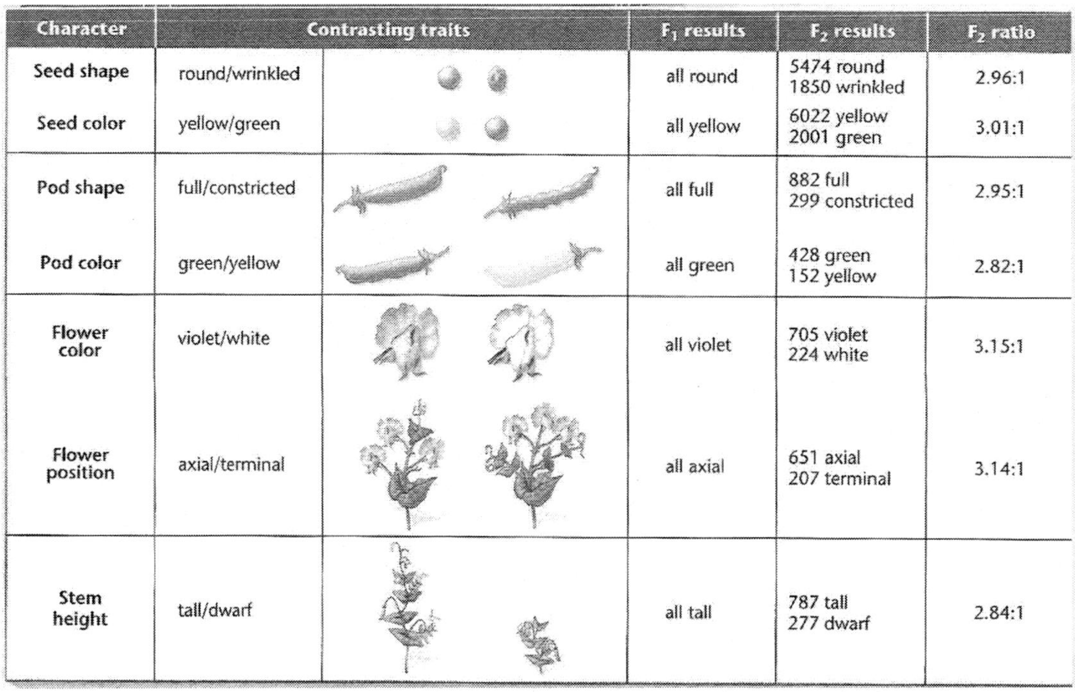

Character	Contrasting traits		F_1 results	F_2 results	F_2 ratio
Seed shape	round/wrinkled		all round	5474 round 1850 wrinkled	2.96:1
Seed color	yellow/green		all yellow	6022 yellow 2001 green	3.01:1
Pod shape	full/constricted		all full	882 full 299 constricted	2.95:1
Pod color	green/yellow		all green	428 green 152 yellow	2.82:1
Flower color	violet/white		all violet	705 violet 224 white	3.15:1
Flower position	axial/terminal		all axial	651 axial 207 terminal	3.14:1
Stem height	tall/dwarf		all tall	787 tall 277 dwarf	2.84:1

Figure 2.4

Parental lines: Round seeds × Wrinkled seeds
↓

F_1: all round
↓

F_2: 3 round:1 wrinkled

Similar results were obtained when Mendel made crosses between plants differing in six other pairs of alternative characteristics. The results of some of these experiments are summarized in Table 2.A.

The important observations were:
1. All F_1 hybrid plants possessed only one of the alternative parental traits.
2. In the F_2 generation, traits of both parents were present.
3. The trait that appeared in the F_1 generation was always present about three times as frequently as the alternative trait in the F_2 generation.

Mendel's Postulates:

Using the consistent pattern of results in the monohybrid crosses, Mendel derived the following four postulates/principles of inheritance.

1. **Unit Factors In Pairs**

The genetic characters are controlled by unit factors that exist in pairs in individual organisms.

2. **Dominance / Recessiveness**

When two unlike unit factors responsible for a single character are present in a single individual, one unit factor is dominant to the other, which is said to be recessive.

3. **Law of Segregation or Law of purity of gametes (1st law of inheritance)**

During the formation of gametes, the paired unit factors separate or segregate randomly so that each gamete receives one or the other.

A Dihybrid Cross - Cross of pea plant showing round and yellow vs wrinkled and green seed characters (Figure 2.3).

Parents:	Round, seeds yellow cotyledons	.	Wrinkled seeds, green cotyledons
Phenotype genotype	WW GG	×	ww gg
	↓		↓
Gametes:	WG		Wg
	↘		↙
F_1 **progeny:**		Ww Gg Round seeds, yellow cotyledons	

Female gametes \ Male gametes	WG	Wg	wG	wg
WG	WW GG	WW Gg	Ww GG	Ww Gg
Wg	WW Gg	WW gg	Ww Gg	Ww gg
wG	Ww Gg	Ww Gg	Ww GG	ww Gg
Wg	Ww Gg	Ww gg	Ww Gg	ww gg

F_2 progeny:	Genotypes		Phenotypes
	1/16 WW GG + 2/16 WWGg + 2/16 Ww GG + 4/16 Ww Gg	=	9/16 round, yellow
	1/16 ww GG + 2/16 ww Gg	=	3/16 wrinkled, yellow
	1/16 WW gg + 2/16 Ww gg	=	3/16 round, green
	1/16 ww gg	=	1/16 wrinkled, green

Plants from a true-breeding line having round and yellow seeds were crossed with plants from a line having wrinkled and green seeds. The F_1 seeds from this cross were round and yellow; that is, they were hybrid for both characteristics or **dihybrid.** If we assume that seed shape and color are independent traits that do not affect one another, this phenotype can be expected from the results of the individual **monohybrid** crosses (Figure 2.4), in which the alleles resulting in round seed shape and yellow seed color were dominant over their respective alternative alleles. The F_2 seeds obtained when F_1 plants were grown and allowed to self-pollinate, had the four possible combinations of phenotypic characteristics with the following frequencies:

Round, yellow	315
Wrinkled, yellow	101
Round, green	108
Wrinkled, green	32
Total:	**556**

Mendel noted that, when the pairs of alternative phenotypes were considered separately, the ratios 423 (315 + 108) round to 133 (101 + 32) wrinkled seeds and 416 (315 + 101) yellow to 140 (108 + 32) green seeds were in each case very close to the 3:1 ratio observed in the F_2 progenies from the monohybrid crosses. He also noticed that the four phenotypes in the F_2 from the dihybrid cross were present in approximately the proportions 9/16 round yellow, 3/16 wrinkled yellow, 3/16 round green, and 1/16 wrinkled green. Similar 9:3:3:1 ratios of F_2 phenotypes were found in the progeny of other dihybrid crosses (see Table 2.A, Figure 2.4).

Mendel recognized that a 9:3:3:1 ratio is expected to result when two independently occurring 3:1 ratios are combined, and formulated the principle of independent assortment.

4. **Law of independent assortment (2nd law of inheritance)**
Segregation of the members of a pair of alleles is independent of the segregation of other pairs in the formation of reproductive cells.

To illustrate, using the dihybrid cross considered, we can represent the dominant and recessive alleles of the pair affecting seed shape as W and w, respectively, and the allelic pair affecting seed color as G and g. Then, the genotype of the F_1 double heterozygote is Ww Gg

The phenotype of the F_1 seeds is round and yellow, indicating that the allele for round, W, is dominant to that for wrinkled, w, and the allele for yellow, G, is dominant to that for green, g.

The result of independent assortment is that W is as likely to be included in a gamete with G as it is with g, and w is equally likely to be included with G or g. Thus, when two pairs of alleles undergo independent assortment, the gametes produced by the double heterozygote are the following:

¼ WG, ¼ Wg, ¼ wG, and ¼ wg

Penetrance, Expressivity, and Pleiotropy

The phenotypic expression of some genes is identical in all organisms with the same genotype. However, the phenotypes determined by most genes are variable. The variation may result from the effects of other genes, or because the biological processes that produce the particular phenotype are sensitive to environmental conditions. Moreover, most genes affect more than one trait. Metabolic pathways are complex and interconnected, and a defect in one enzyme is likely to affect not only the function of the pathway in which it is involved, but also other pathways that interact with it.

The complexities of variable gene expression are considered under the three following categories:

1. **Variable expressivity:** This refers to genes that are expressed to different degrees in different individuals. The different degrees of expression form a continuous series from full expression to almost no expression of the expected phenotypic characteristics. Many genetic diseases in human beings are caused by genes with variable expressivity, and the result is that, some affected persons may be very severely affected, whereas others carrying the same gene are mildly affected.

    Many developmental traits not only fail to penetrate sometimes but also show a variable pattern of expression, from very mild to very extreme, when they do penetrate. For example, cleft palate is a trait that shows both variable penetrance and variable expressivity. Once the genotype penetrates, the severity of the impairment varies considerably, from a very mild external cleft to a very severe clefting of the hard and soft palates.

2. **Incomplete penetrance:** This means that some individuals with a particular genotype do not express the phenotype associated with the genotype. Failure of the phenotype to be expressed may result from the effects of other genes or from environmental conditions. Incomplete penetrance is merely the extreme of variable expressivity, in which expression of the expected phenotype is so mild as to be undetectable. As an example of incomplete penetrance, there are identical human twins in which one twin has a genetically determined abnormality but the other does not. The proportion of individuals whose phenotype matches their genotype for a given character show penetrance of the genotype. A genotype that is always expressed has a penetrance of 100 percent.

3. **Pleiotrophy:** This means multiple phenotypic effects of a single mutant gene. The traits affected have no physiological connection. However, all are secondary consequences of a single genetic defect. Example. Several genetic diseases result in anemia with several symptoms such as lack of energy, easy fatigue, rapid pulse, pounding heart, swelling of ankles, etc.

Co-dominance and Intermediate Inheritance

When both the alleles of a pair are fully expressed in the heterozygote, the genes and the trait are said to be co-dominant. Examples of co-dominance are the various blood groups. A person of blood group AB has both A and B antigens in his red cells, showing that allelic genes A and B are fully expressed and therefore co-dominant.

If a heteterozygote is neither like a homozygote with both the dominant genes, nor like a homozygote with both the recessive genes, the genes concerned and the traits are said to show intermediate inheritance. Sickle-cell anemia is an example of intermediate inheritance. The homozygote for the abnormal allele has severe sickle-cell anemia. The heterozygote for the abnormal allele does not have severe sickle-cell anemia nor is he/she completely normal. A proportion of his/her red blood cells show the sickling phenomenon. Such a heterozygote is intermediate between normal homozygotes and sickle-cell homozygotes; and is said to have the sickle-cell trait.

The term genetic heterogeneity is used to show a condition when more than one inheritance pattern, as well as differences in the degree of clinical manifestations for each of the inherited diseases /varieties is seen. Amelogenesis imperfecta illustrates genetic heterogeneity.

Oligogenic inheritance refers to those characteristics or traits that are inherited by the participation of a few genes. These conditions show greater clinical variation than those inherited through single-gene action. Characteristics such as tooth shape and form, or blood types, are determined by oligogenic inheritance. Many physical characteristics are oligogenic. The various genes that participate in determining a trait can be located in the same chromosome or in different chromosomes.

DROSOPHILA: The Fruit Fly

Before returning to historical developments in human genetics, it is worthwhile to consider briefly the merits of *Drosophila* which has proved to be of great value in genetic research. *Drosophila melanogaster*, possesses several distinct advantages for the study of genetics because

1. It can be bred easily in glass tubes/milk bottles containing ripe banana/ or Drosophila medium in the laboratory.
2. It breeds rapidly and prolifically at a rate of 25–35 generation per annum (8/10 days required for one generation).
3. It has a number of easily recognizable characteristics such as straight / curly wings, red/white eyes and yellow/ebony body which show Mendelian inheritance.
4. *D.melanogaster*, has only four pairs of chromosomes which can be easily identified under the microscope.

In view of the above unique features, fruit flies were used extensively in early breeding experiments by many geneticists and even for the human genome project as model organism along with several other organisms.

Mendelian Inheritance in Man

1. After the rediscovery of Mendel's principles, an early task was to show that they were true for animals and especially for humans.
2. In fact, human families, like the offspring of experimental organisms, show inheritance patterns of both the types discovered by Mendel (autosomal inheritance) and of sex linkage.
3. In general, what in the hand of an experimental geneticist is a mutant phenotype, in the hands of a human geneticist becomes a disease or a condition of disability (mild to severe).

History of Medical Genetics

Mention has been made about the pioneering studies of far-sighted thinkers such as Maupertuis and Adams whose curiosity was aroused by familial conditions such as polydactyly and albinism. John Dalton, observed that some conditions, notably colour blindness and haemophilia, show what is now referred to as sex-or X-linked inheritance, and remarkably even today colour blindness is referred to as *Daltonism*.

The rediscovery of Mendelism in 1901 by Hugo de Vries, Carl Correns, and Erich von Tschermak marked the real beginning of medical genetics and provided an impetus for the study of inherited diseases. Credit for the first recognition of a single gene trait is shared by William Bateson and Sir Archibald Garrod who together proposed that alkaptonuria is due to a rare autosomal recessive gene disorder. In this relatively harmless condition, urine turns dark on exposure to oxygen due to inability on the part of the patient to metabolise homogentisic acid. Garrod (1857–1936) coined the term inborn error of metabolism and demonstrated that four congenital metabolic diseases (albinism, alkaptonuria, cystinuria, and pentasuria are autosomal recessive and suggested that there are biochemical differences among individuals that lead to illness and have a genetic basis. Several hundred such disorders have now been identified giving rise to the field of study known as biochemical genetics.

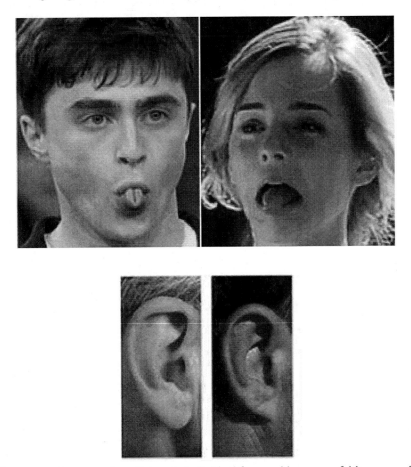

Figure 2.5: Gene expression controls variations in individual features like tongue folding or ear lobe being free or attached, specific to each individual

During the course of the 20th century, it became clear that hereditary factors are implicated in many conditions where different genetic mechanisms are involved. Traditionally, hereditary conditions have been considered under the headings of single gene, chromosomal, multifactorial, and acquired somatic genetic diseases (Figure 2.5). In the past 50 years, a great deal of light has been shed on this area and general human genetics is better understood than in any other organism.

Molecular genetic research has given us powerful tools to study genes. In 1985, Kary Mullis developed a technique called ***Polymerase Chain Reaction*** (PCR), while working for Cetus

Corporation in Emeryville, California – a method that allows researchers to take a minute sample of DNA and amplify it millions of times so that it can be analyzed. Cetus research group soon developed the first thermal cycler which added a new polymerase in each step; this was improved upon by Mullis who suggested the idea of using polymerase isolated from an extremophilic bacterium *Thermophilus aquaticus* to take care of this problem. One application of this technique has been in forensic science, especially disputed parentage including forensic odontology and similar legal disputes. This technique today has translated into a massive gene sequencing process providing huge data and taking human research forward by leaps and bounds.

Classification of Genetic Diseases/Disorders

A) Single Gene Disorders/Single gene defects

Single gene defects are caused by individual mutant genes. The mutation may be present only on one chromosome of a pair (matched with a normal allele on the homologous chromosome) or on both the chromosomes of the pair. Single gene disorders usually exhibit obvious and characteristic pedigree patterns. Such defects however are rare with a frequency of 0.36 and 2.0% for pediatric and general population. Common examples are alkaptonuria, albinism, cystinuria. It was Archibald Garrod who first suggested that albinism and cystinuria could also show recessive inheritance. Soon other examples followed, leading to an explosion in knowledge and disease delineation. By 1966, almost 1500 single gene disorders/traits had been identified prompting the publication of a catalogue of all known single gene conditions by an American human geneticist, Victor Mckusick. By 1994, when the eleventh edition of this catalogue was published, it contained over 6700 entries. On the assumption that there are over 25,000 coding genes in each set of human chromosomes, it is not surprising that the pace of developments in this field, coupled with the need for an up-to-date reference source, has led to the creation of an online version of "McKusick's catalogue". This is known formally as *Online Mendelian Inheritance in Man* (OMIM) and can be accessed *via* the World Wide Web (http://www.ncbi.nlm.nih.gov/omim/). OMIM is written and edited at Johns Hopkins University with input from scientists and physicians around the world. It is a full-text overview of genes and genetic phenotypes that can be used by students, researchers, and clinicians. By the beginning of 1997, OMIM contained a total of 8316 single gene entries; as on June 2001, 17764 genes have been mapped. OMIM home page maintains links to many useful genetic resources including the Genetic Alliance, an umbrella organization of over 600 genetic support groups.

Sequence changes in DNA may be benign in nature giving rise to polymorphic changes that may increase an individual's susceptibility to disease but mutations are the underlying cause of single gene disorders. These disorders may by autosomal or X-linked; they may be dominant if they are expressed in the heterozygous condition or else they are recessive in nature (Tables 2.B and 2.C). The various dominant genes related to phenotypic traits commonly seen in human are: tongue rolling and folding,

Roman nose, absence of sense of smell, while the recessive genes are dimple (freckles) on cheeks, albinism, attached/free ear lobe etc. Although Mendelian disorders are often grouped according to their patterns of transmission, it is perhaps more appropriate to categorize them on the basis of the nature of protein that is affected, because in large part the type of protein affected determines the pattern of inheritance. Hence, in Tables 2.B to 2.D selected single-gene disorders are classified into broad groupings on the basis of the protein abnormality and the various systems involved.

Table 2.B Autosomal Recessive Disorders

System		Disorder
Metabolic	..	➢ Cystic fibrosis
		➢ Phenylketonuria
		➢ Galactosemia
		➢ Homocystinuria
		➢ Lysosomal storage diseases
		➢ α - Antitrypsin deficiency
		➢ Wilson disease
		➢ Hemochromatosis
		➢ Glycogen storage diseases
Hematopoietic	..	➢ Sickle cell anemia
		➢ Thalassemias
Endocrine	..	➢ Congenital adrenal hyperplasia
Skeletal	..	➢ Ehlers- Danlos syndrome (some variants)
		➢ Alkaptonuria
Nervous	..	➢ Neurogenic muscular atrophies
		➢ Friedreich ataxia
		➢ Spinal muscular atrophy

Table 2.C. Autosomal Dominant Disorders

System	Disorder
Nervous	➤ Huntington disease ➤ Neurofibromatosis ➤ Myotonic dystrophy ➤ Tuberous sclerosis
Urinary	➤ Polycystic kidney disease
Gastrointestinal	➤ Familial polyposis coli ➤ von Willebrand disease
Skeletal	➤ Marfan syndrome ➤ Ehlers- Danlos syndrome (some variants) ➤ Osteogenesis imperfecta ➤ Achondroplasia
Metabolic	➤ Familial hypercholesterolemia ➤ Acute intermittent porphyria

Table 2.D. Biochemical Basis and Inheritance Pattern of Some Mendelian Disorders

Protein Type/ Function	Example	Pattern of Inheritance	Disease
Enzyme	Phenylalanine hydroxylase	Autosomal recessive	Phenylketonuria
	β-hexosaminidase		Tay – Sachs disease
	Adenosine deaminase		Severe combined immuno deficiency**
Enzyme Inhibitor	α_1 – Antitrypsin	Autosomal recessive	Emphysema and liver disease
Receptor	Low-density lipoprotein receptor	Autosomal dominant	Familial hypercholesterolemia

Protein Type/ Function	Example	Pattern of Inheritance	Disease
Transport			
Oxygen	Hemoglobin	Autosomal codominant*	α - Thalassemia
			β - Thalassemia
			Sickle cell anemia
Ions	Cystic fibrosis transmembrane conductance regulator	Autosomal recessive	Cystic fibrosis
Structural			
Extracellular	Collagen	Autosomal dominant	Osteogenesis imperfecta; Ehlers-Danlos syndromes**
	Fibrillin	Autosomal dominant	Marfan syndrome
Cell membrane	Dystrophin	X-linked recessive	Duchenne/Becker muscular dystrophy
	Spectrin, ankyrin, or protein 4.1	Autosomal dominant	Hereditary spherocytosis
Hemostasis	Factor VIII	X-linked recessive	Hemophilia A
Growth regulation	Rb protein	Autosomal dominant	Hereditary retinoblastoma
	NF-1 protein	Autosomal dominant	Neurofibromatosis type I

Heterozygotes are either asymptomatic or have mild disease
**some variants are autosomal recessive or X-linked*

As interest in Mendelian inheritance grew, there was much speculation as to how it actually occurred. Walter Fleming (1879) first observed the nucleus in Salamander cells within which there are several thread-like structures called chromosomes, (chroma = colour, soma = body). In 1903, Sutton, a medical student, and Boveri, a German biologist, independently proposed that chromosomes carry the hereditary factors, the genes and proposed the chromosome theory of inheritance.

When the link between Mendelian inheritance and chromosomes was first made, it was thought that the normal chromosome number in humans was 48. However, the correct chromosome number of 46 was established by Tijo and Levan (1956). Shortly thereafter, it was shown that human disorders could be due to loss or gain of a whole chromosome as well as an abnormality in a single gene. Some chromosome abnormalities, such as translocations, are known to run in families and are sometimes said to segregate in a Mendelian fashion.

B) **Chromosome Abnormalities**

In chromosome disorders, the defect is not due to a single mistake/mutation in the genetic blueprint but an excess or deficiency of the genes contained in whole chromosome or chromosomal segments. Improved cytological techniques for studying chromosomes led to the demonstration in 1959 that the presence of an additional number in chromosome 21 (*trisomy* 21) resulted in Down syndrome. As a group, chromosome disorders are quite common, affecting about 7/1000 newborn infants and accounting for about half of all spontaneous first trimester abortions. The identification of chromosome abnormalities has been further aided by the development of various chromosome banding techniques in 1970. These enabled identification of individual chromosomes and helped confirm that loss or gain of even a very small segment of a chromosome can have bad effects on human development.

Recently, it has been shown that several rare conditions featuring mental retardation and abnormal physical features are due to loss of a tiny amount of chromosome material that cannot be detected using a powerful light microscope. These conditions are referred to as microdeletion syndromes and are now being diagnosed using techniques such as FISH (Fluorescent *in situ* hybridisation) which combines conventional cytogenetic chromosome analysis along with newer DNA diagnostic technology of molecular genetics.

C) **Multifactorial Disorders**

Francis Galton, Charles Darwin's cousin evinced interest in human characteristics such as stature, physique, and intelligence. Galton introduced the concept of the regression coefficient as a means of estimating the degree of resemblance between various relatives. This concept was later extended to incorporate Mendel's discovery of (factors) genes to try to explain how characters such as human height and skin colour could be explained by the interaction of many genes, each exerting a small additive effect. This model of quantitative inheritance is now widely accepted and has been adapted to explain the pattern of inheritance observed for several congenital malformations such as cleft lip and palate, diabetes, and hypertension disorders. Recent research has confirmed that multiple genes at multiple loci are involved in several developmental disorders resulting in congenital malformations, disorders of adult life and tend to recur in families but do not show the characteristic pedigree patterns of single trait. Multifactorial conditions are known to make a major contribution to human morbidity and mortality; about 5% in pediatric population while about 60% in the general population.

D) **Acquired Somatic Genetic Disease**

Not all genetic disorders are present from conception. Many billions of cell divisions occur during the course of an average human's lifetime. During each mitosis there is a possibility for the occurrence of both single gene mutations, due to DNA copy errors, and numerical chromosome abnormalities (due to errors in chromosome separation). Accumulation of somatic mutations and chromosome abnormalities are now known to account for a large proportion of malignancy and probably responsible for many other serious illnesses in addition to the process of ageing. Acquired chromosomal aberrations / rearrangements in somatic cells result in loss of critical gene functions and often entire pathways as seen in hematological malignancies. The role of the environment and its various components in driving these processes is very crucial to the understanding of acquired disease.

CHAPTER 3
Chromosome Basis of Heredity

The Boveri–Sutton chromosome theory (chromosome theory of inheritance) identifies chromosomes as the carriers of genetic material where chromosomes are linear structures with genes located at specific sites on them called *loci*. It states that chromosomes seen in dividing cells are passed from one generation to another, which is the basis for inheritance. Sutton worked with grasshoppers to show that chromosomes occur in matched maternal and paternal chromosome pairs that separate during meiosis and thus explained the Mendelian law of heredity.

Waldeyer (1888) proposed the term chromosomes to thread like structures in the cell nucleus. The word chromosome is derived from the Greek word Chroma (=colour) and soma (=body). Chromosomes are considered as being made up of genes. Their behaviour at somatic cell division provides a means of ensuring that the daughter cell retains its own complete genetic complement hence enabling continuity from one generation to the next. Similarly, the behaviour of chromosomes during gamete formation by meiosis enables each ovum and sperm to contain single set of parental genes. The term mitosis was coined by Flemming (1880), derived from the Greek word for "a thread" referring to a chromosome while the term meiosis is derived from the Greek word "to lessen". The reproductive tissue is diploid (2n); the ovaries and testis are characterized by meiosis/reduction division in sex cells to enable them to segregate into haploid (n) sex cells, the ova and sperms. Important features of mitosis and meiosis are summarized in Table 3.A(*i*).

Table 3.A(*i*). Important differences between Mitosis and Meiosis

Features	Mitosis	Meiosis
Location of tissue:	all tissues (somatic) -	only gonadal tissues (ovary/testis)
End products:	diploid somatic cells and growth -	production of haploid sperm/egg cells
Purpose:	growth, repair, asexual reproduction -	sexual reproduction, gene combination
Chromosomes in daughter cells:	same as parent (2n) -	half that of parent(n)
Relationship with daughter cells:	genetically identical -	genetically dissimilar due to recombination
DNA replication/cell division:	one round -	one round of replication; 2 cell divisions
Duration of prophase:	short 30 min (human cells) -	long and complex
Pairing of homologues:	absent -	normally long and complex (Meiosis I)
Recombination:	rare and abnormal -	normally occurs, increases genetic diversity

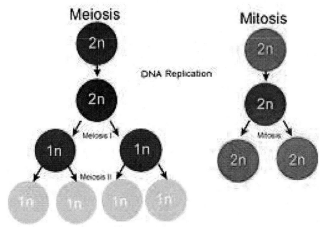

Chromosomes, therefore, are the vehicles which facilitate reproduction and the maintenance of a species. Cytogenetics is the study of chromosomes and their implications in genetics. Most of the knowledge of chromosome structure has been gained using light microscopy. Special stains selectively taken up by DNA have enabled each individual chromosome to be identified. Each chromosome has a centromere that helps in the movement of chromosomes during cell division. Telomere is the tip of the chromosome and maintains its stability and integrity in humans. They consist of many tandem repeats of a TTAGGG sequence which are maintained by the enzyme telomerase. Reduction in level of telomerase and an associated decrease in the number of TTAGGG repeats are believed to be important events in cell death and ageing. In cancers, it works the other way round where there is persistent expression of telomerase and maintenance of telomere length.

Morphologically chromosomes are classified according to the position of the centromere. If located centrally, the chromosome is metacentric, if terminally it is acrocentric, and if an intermediate position, the chromosome is sub-metacentric (Figure 3.1). Acrocentric chromosomes can have appendages called satellites and contain multiple repeat copies of the genes for ribosomal RNA. Homologous pairs are made up of identical partners, referred to as homomorphic chromosomes. An exception are the sex chromosomes, which are of unequal size and are therefore called heteromorphic chromosomes. The numbers of chromosomes possessed by individuals of a species is constant. The diploid chromosome number of several species is shown in Table 3.A*(ii)*.

Table 3.A*(ii)*. Chromosome Numbers In Representative Organisms (most plants and other organisms excluded)

Common name	Genus-Species	Haploid No.	Diploid No.
Cat	*Felis domesticus*	19	38
Cattle*	*Bos Taurus*	30	60
Chicken*	*Gallus domesticus*	39	78
Chimpanzee*	*Pan troglodytes*	24	48
Dog*	*Canis familiaris*	39	78
Frog	*Rana papiens*	13	26
Fruit fly*	*Drosophila melanogaster*	4	8
Pea	*Pisum sativum*	7	14
Grasshopper	*Melanoplus differentialis*	12	24
Horse	*Equus caballus*	32	64
House fly	*Musca domestica*	6	12
Housemouse*	*Mus musculus*	20	40
Human*	*Homo sapiens*	23	46
Mosquito	*Culex papiens*	3	6
Rhesus monkey	*Macaca mulatta*	21	22
Roundworm*	*Caenorhabditis elegans*	6	12

*Model organisms used in Human Genome Project.

Genome: Chromosomes and DNA

Incidentally, it was a professor of botany, Hans Winkler, in 1920, who coined this word genome from 'gene' and 'chromosome' which he used to describe a haploid set of chromosomes in any organism. This word has come to be used as a central term to describe all genetic material in the nucleus and with wide application and technological understanding. There are as many genomes as there are organisms - Prokaryotic, Eukaryotic: Plants, animals, human.

Genomics has become the science of evaluating the normal DNA sequences in the organism by molecular analysis and detailing the regions by genetic mapping, to strive to understand the disease process. The Human genome project was completed in April 2003, two years ahead of schedule, at the National Institutes of Health (NIH) by the National Human Genome Research Institute with an aim of understanding the genetic basis of human health and disease.

Hierarchy of gene organization

Gene – single unit of genetic function
Operon – genes transcribed in single transcript
Regulon – genes controlled by same regulator
Modulon – genes modulated by same stimulus
Element – plasmid, chromosome, phage

Eukaryotic Genome

Eukaryotic genomes are fairly complex and DNA amounts and organization vary widely between species. C value paradox: the amount of DNA in the haploid cell of an organism is not related to its evolutionary complexity or number of genes.

C-value Paradox

Species	DNA bp (C)	Genes	% Coding
phage λ	48,502	67	84
E. coli	4,639,221	4289	85
S. cerevisiae	14,213,386	6241	70
D. melanogaster	180,000,000	18,000	5
Grasshopper	10,000,000,000		
H. sapiens	3,000,000,000	35,000	2-5
Newt	19,000,000,000		~1
Lungfish	140,000,000,000		<1

Drosophila has 20X smaller genome than humans and 2X fewer genes. Newt and lungfish genomes have ~10x and 40x times larger than the human genome.

Chromosome Structure

Chromosomes consist essentially of protein and nucleic acid, and the genetic information is stored in deoxyribonucleic acid (DNA). The DNA in human chromosomes ranges from 14,000 to 73,000 μm in length and extends upto 2 meters.

Chromosomes have been studied under the light microscope for over 100 years. However, it is still imperfectly understood as to how the DNA molecule is packaged with its associated protein into each chromosome. Electron microscope studies have shown that the smallest fibre that can be identified, measures about 10nm in diameter. This is composed of repeating units, called nucleosomes, each consisting of eight histone molecules around which the DNA molecule is coiled, one and three-quarter times. The part of the DNA molecule between nucleosomes is associated with a linker molecule of histone. The linked nucleosomes are in turn coiled into a fibre of 36nm diameter. This is the chromatin fibre that is most readily resolved by examining chromosomes under the electron microscope. It seems that each chromatid has a central scaffold of acidic protein to which the chromatin fibre is attached at regular intervals, and possibly by regions of repetitive DNA, so that loops of chromatin fibre (Laemli loops—each containing about 200000 base pairs) radiate out at right angles to the central scaffold, rather like a bottle-brush. The structure is coiled once more and compacted into a chromatid, which is now visible under the light microscope during cell division. This method of packaging allows the replication and transcription of the DNA molecule in its extended form in the interphase nucleus and also the condensation of the chromosome into a compact structure to ensure its ready passage through cell division (see figure 3.2).

Organization of Eukaryotic Chromosomes

- ✓ **A eukaryotic chromosome contains a long, linear DNA molecule.** A typical chromosome is tens of millions of base pairs in length.
- ✓ **Three types of DNA sequences are required for chromosomal replication and segregation**
- ✓ **Origins of replication** - Origins of replication are interspersed about every 1,00,000 base pairs.
  - **Centromeres** - Centromere forms a recognition site for the kinetochore proteins.
  - **Telomeres** - Telomeres contain specialized sequences located at both ends of the linear chromosome.
- ✓ **Genes are located between the centromeric and telomeric regions along the entire chromosome** (Figure 3.1).
- ✓ **A single chromosome usually has a few hundred to several thousand genes.**
- ✓ **In lower eukaryotes (such as yeast)**
  - Genes are relatively small
  - They contain primarily the sequences encoding the polypeptides
  - Very few introns (intervening sequences between exons) are present and devoid of genes

Coding sequences of a polypeptide (gene-rich)

- ✓ **In higher eukaryotes (such as mammals),**
  - Genes are long
  - They tend to have many introns

40 | Essentials of Human Genetics

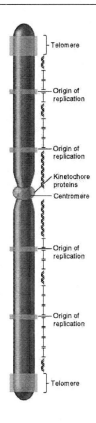

Figure 3.1.

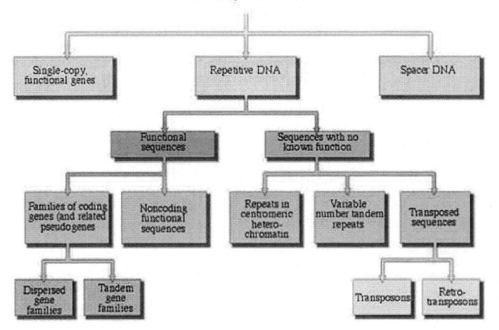

Chromosome Basis of Heredity | 41

Repetitive Sequences - Sequence complexity refers to the number of times a particular base sequence appears in the genome
- There are three main types of repetitive sequences:
  - Unique or non-repetitive – in structural as well as intergenic areas.
  - Moderately repetitive – at origins of replication, transposable elements, genes for rRNA and histones.
  - Highly repetitive – usually non-protein coding, short, 5-100 nucleotide sequences repeated thousand times in a single stretch.

Eukaryotic Chromatin Compaction (Figure 3.2)
✓ If stretched end to end, a single set of human chromosomes will be over one meter long! Yet the cell's nucleus is only 2 to 4 mm in diameter. Therefore, the DNA must be tightly compacted to fit in a cell.
✓ The compaction of linear DNA in eukaryotic chromosomes involves interactions between DNA and various proteins.
Proteins bound to DNA are subject to change during the life of the cell.
These changes affect the degree of chromatin compaction.

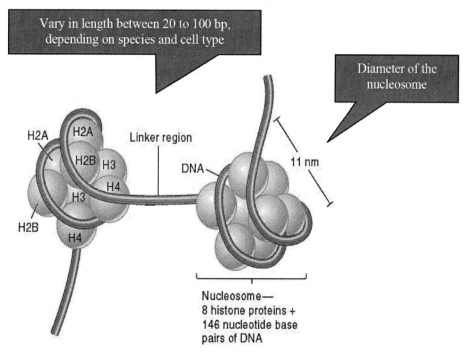

(a) Nucleosomes showing core histones

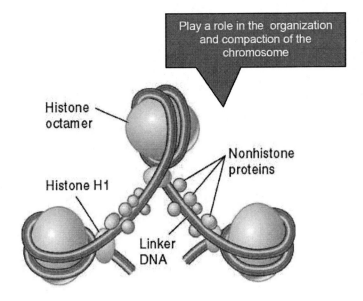

(b) Nucleosomes showing linker histones and nonhistone proteins

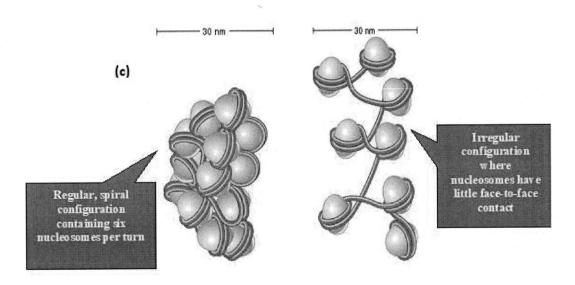

Solenoid model (not correct)

Three-dimensional zigzag model

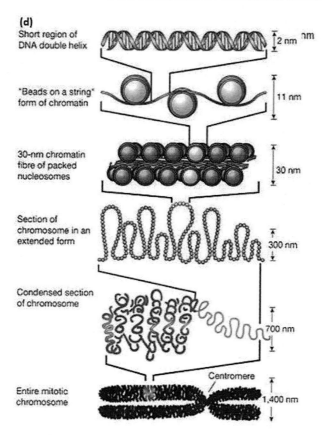

Figure 3.2: (a) Nucleosomes with core histones and linker DNA (b) Linker histones and non-histone proteins associated with nucleosome binding (c) Models showing the nucleosomal configuration to attain a compact structure (d) Chromatin organization into chromosomes.

4 Cytogenetics

CHAPTER

Chromosome Banding

Until about 1970, mitotic chromosomes viewed under the light microscope could be distinguished only by their relative sizes and the positions of their centomeres. The chromosome banding technique was developed by Casperson after staining chromosomes with the DNA binding fluorescent dye, quinacrine mustard. Different regions along the length of each chromosome show a varied intensity of fluorescence so that the various chromosomes could be identified.

Q Banding (Quinacrine banding): This involves the use of fluorescent stains (flourochromes) such as quinacrine hydrochloride or quinacrine mustard which preferentially bind with AT rich DNA. When examined under a fluorescence microscope, each chromosome pair stains in a specific manner of bright and dull bands called the Q bands. This pattern corresponds to that of the G bands.

G Banding (Giemsa Banding) This chromosome banding technique was devised by Mary Lou Pardue and Joe Gall. They found that if chromosome preparations were heat denatured (subject to controlled digestion with trypsin) and then treated with Giemsa stain, they gave a unique staining pattern. See Figure 4.1, Table 4.A.

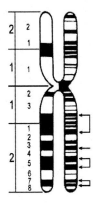

Figure 4.1: G-banded X chromosome

Table 4. A Properties of chromosome bands seen with standard Giemsa

DARK BANDS (G BANDS)	PALE BANDS (R bands)
Stain intensely with dyes that bind, preferentially to **AT** rich regions such as Giemsa and Quinacrine.	Stains weakly with Giemsa and Quinacrine.
May be comparatively rich in **AT** rich.	May be comparatively **GC** rich.
DNAse insensitive.	DNAse sensitive.
Condense early during the cell life cycle but replicate late.	Condense late during cell cycle but replicate early.
Gene poor, genes may be large because, exons are often separated by very large introns.	Gene rich, genes comparatively small because of close clustering of exons.
LINE rich but poor in *Alu* repeats.	LINE poor, but rich in *Alu* repeats.

With various staining procedures, it is now possible to distinguish dark and light bands in metaphase and prometaphase chromosomes under a fairly sophisticated microscope. Each chromosome pair and each chromosome segment of sufficient length has been shown to possess band patterns specific for the respective autosomes and sex chromosomes.

The chromosomes stain dark bands and light bands alternately. The G – bands condense during cell division but replicate late and are DNAse insensitive. The dark bands correspond to bright Q bands. They have majority of lines or bands. G banding shows about 550 bands per haploid genome as standard banding. Starting at the centromere, each chromosome is divided into defined regions and bands. Major subdivisions within cytogenetic bands are numbered. Additional subdivisions are designated using a decimal system. These bands are rich in A-T bases. Pale bands are G negative. Gene poor regions are large, the exons are separated by large introns.

R banding (Reverse banding) The chromosomes are pre-treated with heat in saline/phosphate buffer prior to giemsa, stain weakly with Giemsa and Quinacrine and are DNAse sensitive, resulting in dark and light stained bands (R bands). This pattern is reverse of those produced by Q and G banding. R bands are rich in GC bases and contains more genes. The genes are small with clustering of exons. GC specific chromomycin dyes such as Chromomycin A_3, Oligomycin, mithramycin are used. The technique is useful for identifying deletions or translocations involving the telomeres.

T banding This banding identifies a subset of the R bands which are mostly concentrated at the telomeres. The T bands take intense staining than the R bands and can be seen by giving a severe heat treatment of the chromosomes prior to staining with Giemsa or a combination of dyes and flurochromes. Again, it is good to pick chromosomal rearrangements where telomeres are involved as they stain strongly.

Special Banding Techniques

C banding is thought to demonstrate constitutive heterochromatin. The chromosomes are denatured with saturated solution of Barium hydroxide prior to Giemsa staining. C banding can be done by alkali extraction of DNA from the chromosome. Highly repetitive DNA sequences resist such extraction. C banding can also be done by staining with the AT specific DNA ligand, Hoechst 33258, which produces intense fluorescence of the highly AT rich satellite DNAs found in the C band regions. These techniques stain a small region adjacent to the centromere of all chromosomes and they also stain the distal portion of the Y chromosome. The C bands contain highly repetitive non-transcribed DNA called the heterochromatin. C-banding was earlier used to elucidate the origin of unidentified marker chromosomes or derivative chromosomes.

AgNOR staining is the silver staining of the nucleolar organising regions which are the sites of transcriptionally active ribosomal RNA genes, present on six to eight of the D (three pairs) and G group (two pairs) chromosomes, may be as few as three or on all ten chromosomes (Table 4.B).

Table 4. B Classification of chromosome bands (Sumner 2000)

Class	Principal methods	Other methods
Heteromorphic	Banding	G-11 banding, Q banding, N banding, Distamycin
Euchromatic	Banding	G, Q & R; T banding, various fluorochromes, replication banding
Nucleolus organizer	AgNOR staining	N banding regions (NORs)
Kinetochore	Immunolabelling with autoimmune crest serum	C banding, silver staining, in situ hybridization with alphoid satellite sequences.

Banding techniques and their applications

There are various types of frequently used banding techniques in clinical conditions. They are:
1. **Solid staining:** Although outdated still used for breakage syndromes and fragile sites.
2. **G-banding:** Most widely used for the study of mammalian chromosomes.
3. **Q-banding:** Flourescent staining technique using quinacrine produces similar bands to G banding used for polymorphic variants on chromosomes especially acrocentrics and the Y chromomosome.
4. **C-banding:** This produces dark staining of the constitutive heterochromatin, useful for polymorphic variants of chromosomes.
5. **R-banding:** Reverse of G-banding, unlike G-banding, telomeres stain dark.
6. **NOR staining:** NOR regions contain genes for 18S and 28SRNA, the active transcription sites on chromosomes, useful in identifying small bi-satellited marker chromosomes as in acrocentrics. Silver nitrate is used.

7. **Distamycin banding**: DA-4',6-diamidino-2-phenyl-indole (DA-DAPI) is a very useful technique for identifying small marker chomosomes, fragile sites, also stains constitutive heterochromatic regions. Both DA and DAPI have strong affinity for AT base pairs at similar but not identical sites.

High Resolution banding

In this technique, DNA synthesis in cells is arrested by adding methotrexate to synchronise the dividing cells followed by release of folic acid. The cells are then treated with colchicine to arrest metaphases. The treated cells are harvested in a fixative and stained and the preparations are seen under the microscope. This technique reveals a higher band resolution of 650-800 bands per haploid human genome. The analysis of chromosomes under the microscope (Karyotype analysis) is labour intensive and therefore several automated systems are now employed which find metaphases and arrange the chromosomes as per a standard karyotype. This technique is based on the fact that the human karyotype is made up of chromosomes of different lengths, metaphase chromosomes can also be presented in a flow-cytometry based karyotype which allows sorting of 1000-2000 chromosomes.

Symbols for Chromosomal Nomenclature

There are 46 chromosomes in humans, that is 23 pairs. The first 22 pairs are called autosomes, the last pair of chromosomes is called the sex chromosomes. Any gene on a sex chromosome is referred to as sex-linked. While talking of the chromosomes of *Chrysanthemum*, Shimotomai in 1933 described the symbol 'n' for representing the basic number of chromosomes in a given species. 'Chromosome' is abbreviated to *Chr* after the first use, eg. Chromosome (Chr) 1. The *X* and *Y* chromosomes are indicated by capital letters rather than numbers. The internationally accepted symbols to denote certain abnormal chromosomal features are as follows. Standard abbreviations are followed according to International system for Human Cytogenetic nomenclature 1995, latest being ISCN 2016. Some of them include:

- Sex chromosome abnormalities are described first, followed by autosomal changes in numerical order. Eg. 47,XY,+18 (Male with trisomy 18).
- For each chromosome described, numerical changes are listed before structural abnormalities. Eg.+13,t(13;14).
- Involved chromosome number in parentheses eg. del(2), ins(4).
- If two or more chromosomes are involved in a rearrangement, as with translocation, a semicolon (;) is used to separate chromosome numbers eg. t(2;12)
- Chromosomes abnormalities in cancers also have very definite way of arranging to report the karyotype, where all the clones have to be represented.

Karyotype Karyotype refers to the arrangement of the chromosome set of a somatic cell. It also refers to a photomicrograph of an individual's chromosomes arranged in a standard manner and numbered. The karyotype is characteristic of an individual plant/animal/human/species or genus.

The basis for the arrangement is chromosome size, centromere position, and the specific banding pattern of the chromosome. The karyotype is species specific.

Classification of Chromosomes In humans, there are 22 pairs of autosomes and two X chromosomes in female and X&Y in male. Chromosomes are identified by their length, the position of the centromere, the presence of satellite bodies and other morphological characteristics. It is a standard practice to number the autosomal pairs in decreasing order of chromosome size from 1 to 22 for their classification. The sex chromosomes X and Y retain their distinctive labels. The Denver system of classification was established in 1959 where all the chromosomes including the sex chromosomes were assigned the groups from A to G in order of decreasing chromosome length as shown below.

Group A – Chromosomes 1, 2, and 3
Group B – Chromosomes 4 and 5
Group C – Chromosomes 6 to 12 and the *X* chromosome
Group D – Chromosomes 13 to 15 (the larger acrocentric chromosome with satellite short arms)
Group E – Chromosomes 16 to 18
Group F – Chromosomes 19 to 20
Group G – Chromosomes 21 and 22 (the smaller acrocentrics with satellite short arms) and the *Y* Chromosome

The Paris nomenclature (1971 and 1975) has added more accuracy to the identification of portions of the individual numbered chromosomes. By convention each chromosome arm is divided into regions and each region is subdivided into bands numbering always from the centromere outwards. A given point on a chromosome is designated by the chromosome number, the arm (p or q), the region and the band e.g. 15q12 refers to a band 12 on the long arm of chromosome 15.

A shorthand notation system exists for the description of chromosome abnormalities. Normal male and female karyotypes are depicted as 46,XY and 46,XX respectively. A male with Down syndrome due to trisomy 21 would be represented as 47,XY,+21, whereas a female with a deletion of the short arm of one of the chromosome 5 (*cri-du-chat* syndrome, would be represented as 46,XX,del(5p). A chromosome report reading 46,XY,t(2;4)(p23;q25) would indicate a male with a reciprocal translocation involving the short arm of chromosome 2 at region 2 band 3 and the long arm of chromosome 4 at region 2 band 5. If followed by a decimal point, it represents sub-bands within a dark or a light area.

This system of karyotype nomenclature has also been extended to include the results of FISH studies. For example, a karyotype which reads 46,XX.ish del(15)(qll.2qll.2)(SNRPN-,D15SIO-) refers to a female with a microdeletion involving 15qll.2 identified by *in situ* hybridization analysis defined by probes for the SNRPN and D15SIO locus (D15SIO = DNA from chromosome 15 site 10).

Although human chromosome research has been ongoing for over a century (beginning either with Arnold (1879) or Flemming (1882) or David Hansemann (1891), much of what is used in the basic and clinical work today, has evolved over the past 50 years or so. Tijio and Levan (1956) used cultured fetal lung fibroblasts to determine the correct number of chromosomes in each cell or the karyoptype. Their studies have not only resolved the diploid chromosome number to 46 but established a reliable source for chromosome analysis. However, differentiation between chromosomes remained difficult. Chromosomes could only be identified in 7 gross morphologic groups by size until the 1960s. Chromosome internal structure was better defined by using banding patterns (light and dark bands) created by using special stains. Identification of chromosomes by regions and bands made possible the first descriptions of inherited and acquired genetic changes.

Cytogenetic analysis is an important and integral tool in biomedical scientific studies and has also provided some fundamental insights into the mechanism of human disease (Table 4.C). Historically, staining and analyzing the morphology of chromosomes have provided some of the vital links between the clinical manifestations of the genetic disorders that underlie them. Clinical cytogenetics is routinely used in pre-natal diagnosis and genetic counselling for various diseases. Knowledge of chromosome structure and aberration serves as important beginning to basic and clinical understanding of human disease. Important aspects of study would include:

1. Chromosome structure and its alterations,
2. Cytogenetic (chromosomal) techniques, their interpretation, and nomenclature and
3. Clinical applications of these techniques, with special reference to various diseases in general, congenital and acquired disorders of the head and neck region as well. Syndromes and tumors involving the head and neck region, well-known to the oral and maxillofacial surgeon are linked to chromosomal alterations identified by cytogenetic analysis. Although many craniofacial disorders are believed to result from inherited genetic alteration(s), only a few are associated with gross chromosomal changes demonstrable by karyotypic analysis. Velocardio-facial syndrome (VCFS), also known as Shprintzen syndrome, is a disorder characterized by dysmorphic facial features, cleft palate, cardiac defects, and learning disabilities (Jones, 1988). Frequently, VCFS patients have manifestations of a separate congenital disorder, Di-George sequence (III-IV pharyngeal pouch syndrome). Driscoll *et al* (1992) used a cytogenetic-based approach to show that the disorders share clinical features, because of overlapping chromosomal alterations.

Table 4. C. Flow Chart For Cytogenetic Analysis

Clinical observation (medical and personal history recorded)
Pedigree analysis showing a family history of
particular disease
↓

Obtain tissue specimen
(peripheral blood, bone marrow, tissue biopsies, amniotic fluids and chorionic villi)
↓

Cytogenetic analysis
Chromosome spreads
Chromosome staining
Analyze karyotype for
A] Numeric alterations (gain/loss of chromosomes)
B] Structural alterations
(translocation, insertion, amplification, inversion, deletion)
↓

Further analysis

Prophase/High-resolution cytogenetic analysis
Flow cytometry
Florescent *in situ* hybridisation (FISH)

Cytogenetic analysis has revolutionized our understanding of the chromosomal basis of human neoplasia (Mitelman *et al*, 1997). Although inherited solid tumors of various anatomic sites have been most extensively studied, chromosomal studies with technical advances in cytogenetics, permit the identification of chromosomal alterations of acquired/adult solid tumors such as squamous cell carcinoma of the oral cavity and several salivary gland tumors. Karyotyping of solid tumors has been hampered by technical difficulties that have now been overcome with advanced cytogenetic studies like FISH (Varma and Babu, 1989). First, culturing tissues for analysis is challenging, since tumor cells do not grow, and secondly cancer cells accumulate a multitude of chromosome changes, making the differentiation between primary, pathogenically essential alterations from secondary aberrations difficult. A cytogenetic analysis of salivary gland tumors by Mark et al (1996) illustrates the successes and difficulties of solid tumor analysis. Using G-banding and FISH analysis, they showed several chromosome abnormalities in benign and malignant salivary gland tumors, including translocations, deletions and inversions.

Almost all malignant cells show consistent chromosomal abnormalities that suggest their clonal origin. The number of tumors with abnormal karyotype is continuously updated; for example, the 1994 catalogue of chromosomal aberration in cancer contains information on 3144 different neoplasms with abnormal karyotype by banding analysis.

The gain or loss of genetic material and the presence or absence of growth regulatory genes (oncogenes) are being studied and more than 100 abnormal oncogenes and tumor suppressor genes have been identified. Specific chromosomal deletions have been found in colonic cancer cells that are being used to identify the origin of the metastatic tumor cells. All these studies hope to provide a better understanding of the nature and behavior of these tumors.

Attempts are being made also to use this technique for the detection of precursors or occult colonic adenocarcinormas, and many other cancers. Specific gene translocations are being found in various sarcomas (synovial sarcoma, myxoid liposarcoma, Ewing's sarcoma, rhabdomyosarcoma). In chronic myelogenous leukemia, the c-*abl* oncogene translocates from chromosome 9 to chromosome 22 where the new chr 22 is refered to as 'Philadelphia chromosome' and forms a new oncogenic "hybrid" gene. Listed below are the various conditions other than cancers where a cytogenetic evaluation is warranted.

Common Indications for Cytogenetic Analysis

1. Rule out the classical chromosomal syndromes (e.g. Down syndrome)
2. Multiple congenital anomalies
3. Siblings with chromosomal abnormalities
4. Couple with history of 2 or more fetal losses
5. Abortuses or malformed stillborns
6. Couples with infertility problems
7. Ambiguous genetalia
8. Amenorrhea
9. Pubertal failure in males and females
10. Mental retardation
11. Hematologic disorder
12. Amniotic fluid from mothers of advanced age or history of genetic problems
13. History of chromosome instability syndromes. (e.g., fragile X syndrome)

Molecular Cytogenetics

Flow Cytometry

This technique of modern molecular biology was first developed by Bartholdi et al, 1987. Flow karyotyping is an alternative approach to automated classical karyotype analysis. This procedure exploits the ability of flow cytometry to measure the DNA content of individual chromosomes as they pass in a fluid stream at a speed of upto 2000 per second through the laser beam of a fluorescence-activated cell sorter. Infact the stream of fine droplets has each droplet containing at least one chromosome (as measured by the fluorescence intensity). The droplet containing the chromosomes have a positive charge. The suspension of chromosomes stained by a fluorescent dye (Ethidium bromide), and the fluorescence generated by the laser beam in each chromosome is collected in a photomultiplier tube and stored in a computer. After several minutes, sufficient individual measurements have been collected to generate a histogram or flow karyotype which groups the chromosome measurements according to increasing DNA content. Many chromosomes form separate distinct peaks, and the median of each peak provides an accurate and reproducible measure of the relative DNA content of a particular pair of chromosomes, which is useful in detecting chromosomal deletions and duplications. The flow karyogram has several peaks for the various chromosomes. The area under each peak represents the relative number of chromosomes in each peak, and this has application in the diagnosis of numerical aberrations such as trisomies, eg. Down syndrome.

Chromosome 21 and 22 are almost similar in size and DNA content of chromosome 21 is gene poor and has relatively high percentage of A+T whereas chromosome 22 is gene rich and has a relatively high percentage of G+C chromosome. The size of the X chromosome lies between 7 and 8 chromosomes while the size of the Y chromosome corresponds to chromosome 22.

Another molecular cytogenetic technique is *fluorescent in situ hybridisation* (FISH) which relies on the unique ability of a single stranded DNA (known as a probe) to anneal or hybridise with its complementary target sequence wherever it is located in the genome. The probe is conjugated with a fluorescent label allowing it to be easily seen under ultraviolet beam.

Different types of chromosome specific probes can be used; specific for a centromere or a particular region of a chromosome or a whole chromosome. When whole chromosome paints are used over a metaphase spread, they hybridise to (or paint) all material originating from one or more chromosomes. This technique is useful for complex chromosomal rearrangement and in identifying the nature of aberrant chromosome material if any. As a corollary, an additional portion of unidentified chromosome material can be extracted using a cell sorter. This can be amplified using polymerase chain reaction (PCR) and used as a probe for hybridisation to a normal metaphase spreads.

FISH technique is also used in interphase nuclei for rapid diagnosis in syndromes like trisomy 21 especially in prenatal testing. The technique is also preferred when testing leukemic blood or bone marrow for specific chromosomal rearrangements with targeted therapies or indicating particular type of prognosis.

Chromosome Painting

Flourescent labeling of whole chromosome by a FISH procedure involves labeled probes each consisting of complex mixture of different DNA sequences from a single chromosome, a technique which was developed in the late 1980s. At that point of time, flow-sorted chromosome libraries were used for the purpose. Currently, a large number of copies of DNA from each of these chromosomes are obtained by putting them into bacterial cells to amplify them. Later these fragments of DNA are fluorescent-labeled with differently coloured label (chromosome paints) that hybridise to metaphase chromosomes/interphase cells, thereby giving results as spectral karyotyping (Dauwerse et al, 1992). Nederlof (1989) showed that probes could be detected using hapten/affinity reagent systems with the fluorochromes amino methyl coumarin acetic acid, fluorescein isothiocyanate (FITC) and tetra methyl rhodamine isothiocyanate (TRITC); later on, varying ratios of the three fluorochromes generated different identifiable colours that could be used to detect sufficient targets. Simultaneous hybridisation of multiple chromosomes with differently florescent labeled probes is possible at the same time. This technique has wide applications in cancer cytogenetics. The origin of un-identified chromosome material is revealed by the chromosome to which it hybridizes and is called as reverse painting, a technique also good to identify de-novo chromosome duplications.

5 Molecular Genetics

CHAPTER

Miescher (1869) first isolated a unique molecule, nuclein which was DNA and proteins, a substance made up of hydrogen, oxygen, nitrogen and phosphorus. The existence of nuclei acids as genetic material, capable of replication, storage, expression, and mutation came from several studies of transformation in bacteria and their bacteriophages.

The central dogma of molecular biology is that genetic information flows from DNA to RNA during chromosome replication and from DNA to protein during gene expression. The flow of information from DNA to protein occurs in two steps:
1) Transcription of DNA to RNA, and
2) Translation of RNA to protein.

WATSON-CRICK MODEL OF DNA

1) Two right-handed helical polynucleotide chains are coiled around a central axis and has deoxyribose sugar and phosphate backbone (Figure 5.1).
2) The double helix axis measures 20 A° in diameter.
3) Each complete turn of the helix is 34 A° long and has 10 base/ pairs each per turn.
4) In any segment of the molecule, alternating larger major grooves and smaller minor grooves are apparent along the axis.
5) The two chains are antiparallel i.e. C-5' to C-3' orientations and run in opposite directions.
6) The bases of both chains are flat, lying perpendicular to the axis i.e. they are stacked on one another, 3-4 A° apart and are located on the inside of the structure.
7) The nitrogenous bases of opposite chains are paired to one another as the result of formation of hydrogen bonds. i.e. Adenine pairing with Thymine and Guanine with Cytosine and this is important genetic concept of complementarity.
8) Two forms of DNA i.e. left-handed (Z-DNA) and right-handed (B-DNA) occur, the latter is common.

9) Watson, Crick, and Wilkins were awarded the Noble prize in medicine in 1962 for this outstanding remarkable and significant contribution to biology and medicine.

Watson and Crick (1953) suggested that the replication of double helix could take place by unwinding of the DNA, so that each strand would form a newly synthesized strand. For example, when a double helix is unwound at an adenine-thymine (A-T) base pair, one unwound strand would carry A and the other would carry T. During replication, the A in the template DNA would pair with T in a newly replicated DNA strand giving rise to an A-T base pair. T in the other template strand would pair with A in the other newly replicated strand giving rise to another A-T base pair. Thus, one A-T base pair in one double helix would result in two A-T base pairs in two double helices. This process would repeat at every base pair in the double helix of the DNA molecule.

This mechanism is called semiconservative replication because although the centre double helix is not conserved in replication, each strand in every daughter DNA molecule has an intact template strand and an intact newly replicated strand (Figure 5.2).

Classification of Nuclear DNA

1. Unique with non-repetitive sequence DNA constituting 60 to 70% of genome. This is the structural gene. It also transcribes heterogenous RNA & precursor of transfer and ribosomal RNA.
2. Repetitive sequences are present mainly in Q and G bands and it is presumed that in man most of the abnormalities occur with large amount of such moderately repetitive sequences.

Classification of DNA

1. **Nuclear DNA (nDNA)**
    - With repetitive sequence 30-40%, mainly satellites.
    - With non-repetitive sequence of genes, 60-70%, single or low copy number.
2. **Mitochondrial DNA (mt DNA)**
    - Circular, responsible for cytoplasmic inheritance and carries number of genes which affect maternal genome (mitochondrial inheritance) with various types of diseases.
3. **Recombinant DNA (rDNA)**
    - Hybrid form of DNA produced by inserting a gene or part of gene from one organism into genome of another organism.
4. **Chloroplast DNA (cp DNA)**
    - Circular, present in chloroplast of plants and carries genes responsible for photosynthesis in plants.

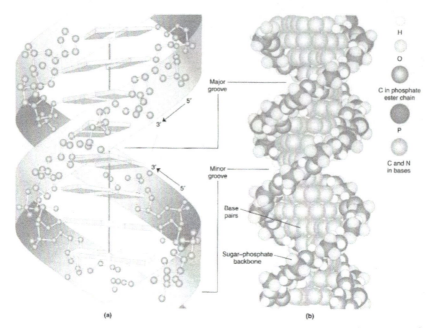

Figure 5.1: (a) The ribbon diagram of DNA showing staking of base pairs (b) Shows the major and minor grooves

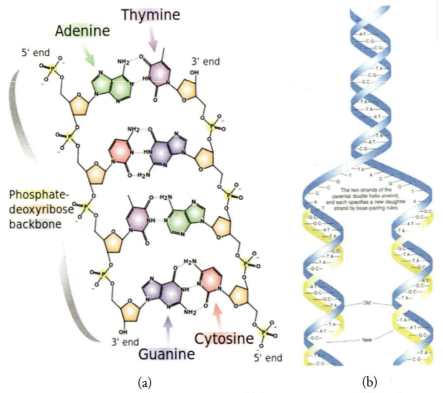

Figure 5.2: (a) Nucleotides comprising the DNA structure (b) Semi conservative DNA replication

Chromosomal DNA

DNA in a chromosome is packed in such manner so as to be easily available. Equal amounts of DNA and a protein – histone, combine in a chromosome. A human diploid cell nucleus contains about 6×10^9 µm base pairs of DNA and 3000 base pairs are present in a length of 1 micron, the total length of DNA per nucleus is 2×10^6 µm i.e. 2 meters while nucleus itself is not more than 10µm in diameter. The human genome contains about 2.7×10^9 nucleotide pairs which can code for about three million genes. Out of these, only 30,000 structural genes are formed by transcription and translation. The function of remainder of DNA is not known. The largest chromosome, chromosome 1 has about 8000 genes and the smallest has about 300 genes.

The secondary constrictions of the five pairs of acrocentric chromosomes carry the genes for 18S and 28S ribosomal RNA. The gene for synthesis of 5S ribosomal RNA is situated near the ends of longer chromosomes. These nucleolar organiser regions are important in the formation of the nucleolus during interphase. In the following metaphase, the dissolution of the nucleolus happens and yet some of these acrocentrics may be mildly associated at their satellites called satellite association. The frequent non-disjunction abnormalities in these chromosomes give rise to Robertsonian translocations.

Triple DNA

It is well known that DNA is double-stranded and RNA is single-stranded. However, it has been known that RNA can be triple-stranded. A surprising discovery of triple DNA also called as ***triplex DNA*** or H-DNA has been made by Rich et al. in the late 1950s *in vitro*. In this, the third strand binds to the other two, by specific base pairing and it can be used to recognize a specific DNA sequence (Figure 5.3). The base pairing rules are rather different.i.e. a thymine in the synthetic DNA will bind near a A-T pair in the biological DNA, and that a cytosine in the synthetic DNA will bind near a G-C pair. The biological significance of Triplex DNA is not fully known but it can be used as a DNA probe or to block gene activity. In the latter, a short oligonucleotide is made that binds to a gene, thereby preventing the RNA polymerase from opening it and copying it onto RNA. This has the same effect as on antisense agent made against the gene product, but it acts at the DNA level. The work on this is limited but has application in aptamer (short length DNA molecules selected to bind to a target amino acid and not DNA) technology. This is somewhat similar to DNA motifs. Binding of a third strand to the double helix is also possible in left-handed DNA called the Z-DNA. This structure occurs naturally in gene promoters. The third strand binds to a B-form DNA double helix by forming Hoogsteen base pairs or reversed Hoogsteen hydrogen bonds.

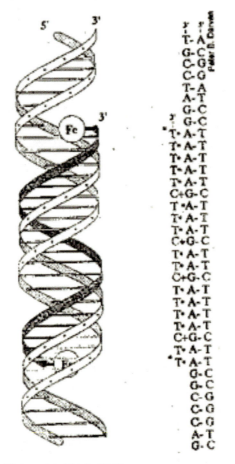
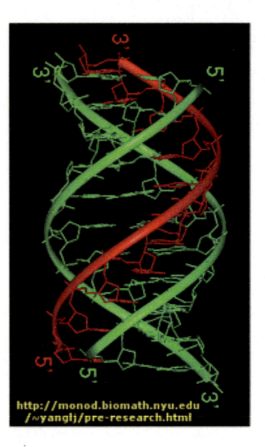

Figure 5.3: Triple DNA structure

RIBONUCLEIC ACID (RNA)

RNA differs from DNA basically in three respects:
1) It has ribose sugar in place of deoxyribose sugar of DNA.
2) Of the four bases three are common in DNA and RNA. They are Adenine, Cytosine, and Guanine. The fourth base in DNA is Thymine and in RNA, it is Uracil.
3) RNA molecule is usually single-stranded while DNA has two strands.

RNAs are of the following types:
1. **mRNA** - messenger RNAs carry information from DNA to ribosomes.
2. **tRNA** - transfer RNA - small molecules work as adaptors between amino acids & codons on mRNA during translation.
3. **rRNA** - ribosomal RNA - components of ribosomes translate nucleotide sequence of mRNA into amino acids.

4. **Sn-RNA** -small nuclear RNA
5. **mi-RNA**-micro RNA
6. **TRNA**- Toxic RNA

Information moves from DNA to the ribosomes where proteins are synthesized. Transfer RNAs (tRNA) are small RNA molecules that function as adaptors between amino acids and the codons in mRNA during translation. Ribosomal RNAs (rRNAs) are structural components of the ribosomes, the intricate machines that translate nucleotide sequences of mRNAs into amino acid sequences of polypeptides. Small nuclear RNAs (snRNA) are structural components of spliceosomes, the nuclear structures that excise introns from nuclear genes.

There are one to four tRNAs for each of the 20 amino acids specified by the genetic code. The tRNA molecules are 70 to 90 nucleotide long and fold into clover leaf-shaped structures by intramolecular base-pairing. In its folded form, each tRNA has a specific amino acid attached at one end and a triplet nucleotide sequence called the anticondon at the other end. The recognition of nucleotide sequences in mRNAs by tRNAs is mediated by base-pairing between the anticodon in the tRNAs and the codon in the mRNA.

Ribosomal RNAs are essential components of ribosomes. The ribosomal RNAs interact with over 50 different ribosomal proteins to produce the complex three-dimensional structure of the ribosome. Eukaryotic ribosomes are more complex than those of prokaryotes; they contain four rRNAs designated 5s 5.8s, 18s and 28s rRNA that are approximately 120, 160, 1900, and 4700 nucleotide in length, respectively.

Five different small nuclear RNAs are present in spliceosomes. As the name implies, they are small in size ranging from 100 to 215 nucleotides long in mammals. Unlike the other RNAs, snRNAs never leave the nucleus. Instead they interact with about 40 nuclear proteins to form spliceosomes, and they play key roles in the excision of non-coding sequences from the transcripts of nuclear genes to form mature mRNA.

All types of RNA-mRNA, tRNA, rRNA, and snRNA-are produced by transcription. Unlike mRNAs which specify polypeptides the final products of tRNA, rRNA, and snRNA genes are RNA molecules, that is transfer RNA, ribosomal RNA, snRNA molecules are not translated.

THE GENETIC CODE

It was evident that genes control the structure of polypeptides. The attention of molecular biologists was then focused on how the sequence of the four different nucleotides in DNA could control the sequence of the 20 amino acids present in proteins. With the discovery of the mRNA intermediary, the question became one of how the sequence of the four bases present in mRNA molecules could specify the amino acid sequence of polypeptides. What is the nature of the genetic code relating mRNA base sequences to amino acid sequences? Clearly the symbols or letters used in the code must be the bases; but what comprises a codon the unit or word specifying one amino acid or actually one aminoacyl- tRNA?

Properties of the Genetic Code: An Overview

The main features of the genetic code were worked out during the 1960s. Cracking the code was one of the most exciting areas in the history of science, with new information reported almost daily. By mid-1960s the genetic code was largely solved. The most important properties are

1. *The genetic code is composed of nucleotide triplets.* Three nucleotides in mRNA specify one amino acid in the polypeptides product; thus each codon contains three nucleotides and is linear.
2. *The genetic code is unambiguous* that each triplet specifies for a single amino acid.
3. *The genetic code is non-overlapping.* Each nucleotide in mRNA belongs to just one codon except in rare cases where genes overlap.
4. *The genetic code is comma-free.* There are no commas or other forms of punctuation within the coding regions of mRNA molecules. During translation, the codons are read consecutively.
5. *The genetic code is degenerate.* All but two of the amino acids and codons for amino acids are specified by more than one codon.
6. *The genetic code is ordered.* Multiple codons for a given amino acid and codons for amino acids with similar chemical properties are closely related, usually differing by a single nucleotide.
7. *The genetic code contains start and stop codons.* Three codons UAG, UAA, UGA do not code for amino acids but act as terminator codon signals.
8. *The genetic code is universal to all forms of life.*

NUCLEOTIDE SEQUENCE COMPOSITION

Eukaryotic organisms including man differ widely in the proportion of the genome consisting of repetitive DNA sequences and in the types of these sequences that are present. A eukaryotic genome typically consists of three components:

1. **Unique or single-copy, sequence**. This is usually the major component and typically forms 30 to 75 percent of the chromosomal DNA in most organisms.
2. **Highly repetitive sequences.** This component constitutes from 5 to 45 percent of the genome. Some of these sequences are the satellite DNA referred to earlier. The sequences in this class are typically from 5 to 300 base pairs per repeat and are duplicated as many as 10^5 times per genome. Alu family is characteristic of mammals
3. **Middle repetitive sequences.** This component is from 1 to 30 percent of a eukaryotic genome and includes sequences that are repeated from a few times to 10^5 per genome.

These different components can be identified according to the number of bands that appear in Southern blots with the use of appropriate probes.

Nuclear Genes

It is estimated that there are up to 20,000 genes in the nuclear genome which code for specific proteins in humans, and almost an equal number of them that do not encode proteins. The distribution of these genes varies greatly between different chromosomes and certain chromosomal regions, with heterochromatic and centromeric regions containing few and the majority being located away from the centromere and in sub-telomeric regions.

Many human genes are single copy genes coding for polypeptides which carry out a variety of cellular functions. These include enzymes, hormones, receptors, and structural and regulatory proteins. Many genes have similar functions having arisen through gene duplication events with subsequent evolutionary divergence. Some are found together in clusters, while others are dispersed throughout the genome constituting what are known as multigene families.

Multigene families

Multigene families can be split into two types, classical gene families which show a high degree of sequence homology and gene super families which have limited sequence homology but are functionally related. Multigene families can be physically close together, e.g. the α- and β-globin gene clusters on chromosomes 16 and 11.

Classical gene families

Examples of classical gene families include the numerous copies of genes coding for the various ribosomal RNAs which are clustered as tandem arrays at the nucleolar organizing regions on the short arms of the five acrocentric chromosomes and the different transfer RNA gene families which are located in numerous clusters interspersed throughout the human genome.

Gene superfamilies

Examples of the gene superfamilies are the HLA genes on chromosome 6 and the T cell receptor genes which have structural homology with the immunoglobulin genes. It is believed that these are almost certainly derived from duplication of a precursor gene with subsequent evolutionary divergence.

Gene structure

The original concept of a gene as a contiguous sequence of DNA coding for a protein was turned on its head in the early 1970s by detailed analysis of the structure of the β-globin gene which revealed it to be much longer than the length necessary to code for the β-globin protein. The gene was found to contain non-coding intervening sequences or introns separating the coding sequences or exons. It appears to be the exception for genome in jawed vertebrates like humans and mice to consist of non-coding intronic sequences within the nuclear genes.

The number and size of introns in various genes in humans are extremely variable, although there is a general trend that the larger the gene, the greater the number of exons. Individual introns can be far larger than the coding sequences and some have been found to contain coding sequences for other genes, i.e. genes occurring within genes. 25% of the human genome may be containing intronic sequences.

C-myc is an oncogene on chromosome 8 which encodes for a nuclear binding protein that stimulates cell division. The inappropriate expression of c-myc protein, usually brought about by structural aberrations in the gene's anatomy, is associated with a number of human malignancies.

Figure 5.4 is a schematic diagram of chromosome 8 as it would appear in a Giemsa-stained metaphase karyotype. The light-and dark-staining bands on the short (p) and the long (q) arms of the chromosome define physical areas on the chromosome. The location of c-myc on the long arm at 8q24.21 is indicated below.

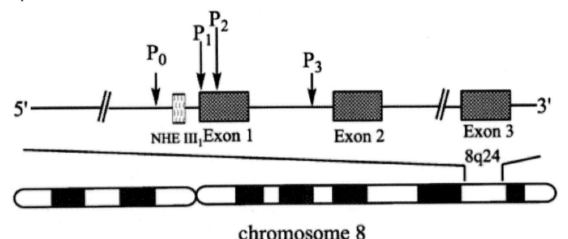

Image courtesy: Chen et al, 2014. Int J Biol Sci.

Figure 5.4 The genomic structure of c-myc.

C-myc is a small gene, consisting of three exons and spanning only 5,000 base pairs. This is a distance of 0.005 centiMorgans. The spacing between exons 1 and 2 of the c-myc gene is 1,616 base pairs, and between exons 2 and 3 the spacing is about 1,300 base pairs. Important structures within the myc gene are indicated in Figure 5.4. Pl and P2 are two promoters which help control the expression of this gene. A promoter is a region associated with a gene which regulates gene expression. There are other regulatory elements associated with genes besides promoters. For example, the c-myc gene has two TATAA boxes, near exon 1. TATAA boxes are also regulators of gene initiation. C-myc is unusual as a gene in that exon 1 contains no codons for the c-myc protein, but exon 1 apparently has a regulatory function. Coding for the protein begins with the ATG sequence 16bp from the start of exon 2 and continues through the second and most of the third exon. At the end of the third exon are coding sequences for a poly A tail common to the end of most messenger RNA molecules. The intron sequences between exons 2 and 3 are initially transcribed into RNA but are then spliced out before the final messenger RNA molecule is exported to the cytoplasm. The c-myc messenger RNA is approximately 2,300 bp long and codes for a protein of 439 amino acids.

The entire base-pair sequence for c-myc is known for humans and several non-human species. There are very few differences in the genomic structure of c-myc between species. This is the case in general for oncogenes which are highly conserved in terms of their structure throughout evolution. The complete DNA sequence for the second exon of the c-myc oncogene is shown in Figure 5.5. Let us look at the detailed structure of the gene as represented in this sequence data. Despite the fact that exon 2 starts at codon CAG, it is not until the codon ATG which codes for methionine that marks the the initiation codon for RNA to protein translation. The second exon of c-myc terminates with the codon TCA, which codes for the amino acid serine, and is where starts the second intron that spans more than 1,300 base pairs.

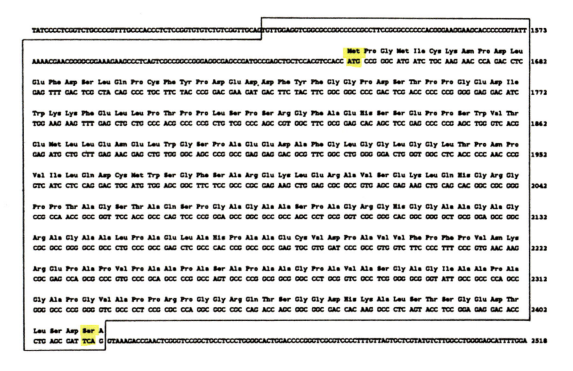

Figure 5.5 Exon2 sequence of c-myc gene Highlighted areas show CAG at the start point whereas ATG is the start codon to translation initiation. Exon 2 terminates with a TCA which codes for amino acid Serine.

The DNA sequence data for the c-myc oncogene shows some of the challenges faced by the human genome project or faced by any lab dealing with DNA sequencing data. The raw data for DNA sequencing are derived from an autoradiograph of a sequencing gel. A typical sequencing gel can decode 200-500 base pairs. As DNA sequence data are acquired, they must be analyzed. Until the entire sequence for a gene is assembled, we do not know where a particular stretch of DNA base pairs "fits in." To analyse DNA sequence data, we first look for an open reading frame. An open reading frame is a series of base pairs in which the stop codons are not encountered for a long stretch. We know that DNA sequences are read three letters at a time by the protein translating machinery. Three codons UAG, UAA, and UGA are called stop codons, because they specify a stop to the translation of RNA into protein. A stop codon is like a period at the end of a sentence. In searching for an open reading frame we have an additional problem in that we do not have a frame of reference in which to begin. We do not know at which letter to start, since we are in the middle of the message. To search for an open reading frame, we try all three of the possible reading frames. We begin at the first base pair and read in groups of three, then shift to the second base pair and read in groups of three, and finally shift to the third pair.

DNA DIAGNOSIS

Recombinant DNA (r-DNA) techniques have enhanced our understanding of the structure & function of human genes. r-DNA technology has application in clinical genetics (DNA-Diagnosis). The following are some important useful techniques:

1) **Southern Blot Technique:** This involves gel electrophoresis with the use of specific probes. This technique is labour intensive (7-14 hours) and involves use of radio-active material hence requires safety precautions. The sequence of steps is as follows-
   5-10µg DNA from WBC is taken and treated with Restriction Enzyme resulting in sequence specific cuts of DNA-fragments. These are separated by gel electrophoresis and the denatured DNA is transferred to membrane. Radio-labelled DNA probe is added. The probe recognizes and hybridizes with complementary DNA sequence thus allowing the specific fragment of interest to be detected.

2) **Polymerase Chain Reaction: (PCR)** This involves rapid amplification of target DNA/RNA sequences. This technique is sensitive, specific and speedier, therefore has revolutionized genetic analysis and detection of disease (e.g. Sickle cell disease etc). PCR is important because of its efficiency and therefore routinely used in detection of diseases. 1µg or a single cell is enough for PCR hence for DNA fingerprinting in criminology, this method is very useful as also in cases of disputed paternity.

3) **Allele Specific Oligonucleotide (ASO) probe analysis:** This technique uses two synthetic oligonucleotide probes, one specific for a known genetic mutation, the other specific for a known normal sequence of the same region. The ASO probes for the normal and mutant genes are used as hybridisation probes to determine whether a patient has 2 copies of normal gene or has a mutation responsible for a particular disease.

4) **Electrophoresis of single stranded DNA:** This technique allows the identification of differences between DNA sequences from a patient with a particular disease and from a normal control

person. The differences are detected by shifts in the bands that are seen in the electrophoretic bands.

5) **DNA sequencing:** This is the more precise method to characterise a segment of DNA in order to obtain the exact sequence of DNA. Abnormal mutations are identified and then used to detect such mutations in family members. Now is the era of DNA diagnostics for human disease using next-generation sequencing (NGS) where the whole genome or whole exome is sequenced to identify mutations specific to disease in an individual. The technique is also used for targeted exome sequencing for instance, in cancers, to identify genomic alterations which can charecterize the disease better and also for using these findings as targets for molecular therapies.

Apart from the above techniques there are some more techniques used in DNA diagnosis where point mutations (Tay Sachs disease), major gene rearrangements & conditions like thalassemia and Duchenne muscular dystrophy, Becker Muscular dystrophy are diagnosed.

Applications

1. DNA finger printing is now widely used all over the world in forensic science for example as in **Forensic odontology.**
1. Genetic disorders are easily recognised before their clinical onset.
2. In transplantation, tissue matching is essential and uses these methods.
3. The human genome project routinely relies on this technique to locate genes on various chromosomes.

DNA BANKING

- DNA banking is a relatively new concept. DNA banks store DNA from crucial relatives in an effort to ensure that no family members will be denied DNA testing due to lack of available DNA
- This is done by extracting DNA from any tissue usually white blood cells. For large supply, the WBCs are immortalised after exposure to the Epstein Bar virus which allows the cells to grow for few weeks so that unlimited supply of DNA is possible.
- DNA banking is also done by storing semen / eggs / tissues at ultra low temperature.

6

CHAPTER

Mutations

The term mutation is derived from the Latin word 'Mutare', to change. Hugo de Vries, one of the rediscoverer of Mendelism described mutations as inherited variations in his "***Die Mutation Theorie***". Mutation may occur anywhere in the genome, specific to particular chromosome, the chromosome segment is defined accordingly and even the gene bearing the mutation is identified, to be used in diagnosis. Mutations may be spontaneous (natural; with no specific agent due to errors in DNA replication) or can be induced by radiations or some chemical agent called mutagen. Mutations may be somatic (somatic tissue) or gametic (germinal). Mutations in somatic cells are not transmitted but are important in the causation of cancers, aging process and some neurodegenerative conditions. Mutation rate/frequency is very low from gene to gene within a species or from organism to organism.

Characteristics of mutant genes

1. They occur in small range.
2. Mutant genes are restricted to specific loci.
3. Mutant gene can back mutate (Reverse mutation).
4. Neighbouring loci are unaffected.

Naming the mutant gene

1. Mutant genes are named according to the most prominent character produced eg. albinism.
2. Genes with effect on more than one character/phenotype will have pleiotropic effects.

Kinds of mutations

1. Detrimentals constitute 8% with no visible effect.
2. Lethals constitute 20% causing death in homozygote.
3. Visible constitute 1% detectable with visible phenotype.

4. May be autosomal recessive / dominant.
5. May be sex-linked recessive.

Classically, there are two sources of genetic variation: **chromosomal mutations** and **gene mutations.** The former, also called **chromosomal aberrations,** includes duplication, deletion, or rearrangement of chromosome segments. Gene mutations result from a change in the stored chemical information in the DNA sequence. Such a change may include substitution, duplication, insertion or deletion of nucleotides. Mutations may affect behaviour patterns of an organism, for example, circadian rhythms of animals may be altered. The primary effect of **behaviour mutations** is difficult to discern. For example, the mating behaviour of a fruitfly may be impaired if it cannot beat its wings. However, the defect may be in: (1) the flight muscles, (2) the nerves leading to them, or (3) the brain, where the nerve impulses that initiate wing movements originate.

Biochemical mutations in humans are best exemplified by hemophilia and sickle-cell anemia. Such mutations are not visible and do not affect morphology but have a general effect on the well-being and survival of the affected person.

Still another type of mutation may affect the regulation of genes. A regulatory gene may produce a product that controls the transcription of another gene. In other instances, a region of DNA either close to or far away from a gene may modulate its activity. In either case, **regulatory mutations** may disrupt target gene activity and permanently activate or inactivate a gene. Knowledge of genetic regulation depends on the study of mutations that disrupt this process.

Another group consists of **lethal mutations**. Nutritional and biochemical mutations also fall into this category. Various human biochemical disorders, such as Tay-Sachs disease and glycogen storage disorders may be lethal at different points in the life cycle of humans. Based on the effects they generate on the DNA sequence, their source, mutations are characterized differently (Figure 6.A).

Physical Mutagenesis

Ultra-violet and high energy radiations are two components of physical mutagenesis. Both are part of the electromagnetic spectrum and have shorter wavelengths; X-rays and γ-rays are much shorter and high energy radiations capable of ionizing DNA and hence generating mutation.

Ultra-violet rays have a wavelength of 260nm and affect pyrimidines, forming thymine dimers. *Xeroderma pigmentosum*, a rare autosomal recessive disorder in humans, predisposes individuals to epidermal pigment abnormalities. Exposure to sunlight results in malignant growth of the skin. James Cleaver (1968) showed that cells from Xp patients were deficient in the unscheduled DNA repair elicited in normal cells by ultraviolet light exposure. In 1974, the presence of low levels of photoreactivating enzyme in Xp cells connected with the disease was established.

Muller (1927) working with *Drosophila* showed that X-rays penetrate cells, electrons are ejected from the atoms of molecules encountered by the radiation and cause chromosome breaks. A linear relationship between X-ray doses and the induction of mutation had been established. For each doubling of dose twice as many mutations are induced. These observations may be interpreted in the form of Target theory proposed by Crowther and Dessaner (1924) who propose that there are one or more sites or targets, within cells and that a single event of irradiation at one site will bring about a damaging effect, or mutation. In other words, the target theory says that one, 'hit' of irradiation will cause one event or mutation when the X-rays interact directly with the genetic material. Ionising radiations interact with water releasing highly reactive ions, called the free radicals which react with DNA resulting in mutagenic effect. The frequency of mutations by X-rays is proportional to the radiation dose. The mutagenic and lethal effects of ionizing radiations at low to moderate doses result in three types of damage to DNA, viz,

1. single stranded breakage in sugar-phosphate backbone which are efficiently repaired.
2. double stranded breakage and
3. alterations in nucleotide sequences, which cause mutations and lethality. In eukaryotes ionising radiations result in chromosome breakage.

Genetic effects

Experiments with animal and plant systems have shown that the number of mutations produced by irradiation is proportional to the dose; the larger the dose the more the mutations produced. It is believed that there is no threshold below which irradiation has no effect, i.e. even the smallest dose of radiation can produce a mutation. The genetic effects of ionising radiation are also cumulative so that each time a person is exposed to radiation, the dose received has to be added to the amount of radiation already received. The total number of radiation-induced mutations is directly proportional to the total grand dose.

The genetic effects of radiation may not be manifested in the generation which is exposed to radiation but may appear only in subsequent generations. If a dominant mutation is produced then it will be manifest in the next generation, but a recessive mutation will only be manifest if two heterozygotes with a mutation in the same gene have children. If a recessive mutant allele is very rare then the chance of this happening will be small. It was argued, however, that recessive mutations induced on the X chromosome would be immediately manifest in hemizygous male offspring of mothers who had been irradiated. If these mutants were lethal then the number of male births would be diminished; the sex ratio (number of male births divided by the number of female births) would be reduced. If X-linked dominant lethal mutations were produced then there would be an equal chance of both male and female babies being eliminated and the sex ratio would remain unchanged. Recessive X-linked lethal mutations would lead to an excess of live male births with a resultant increase in the sex ratio.

It is now known that a radiation dose of 50-150r is lethal to 50% of human cells in culture. Whole body radiation of 400r is fatal to individuals and 100r is sufficient to cause radiation sickness. Sub-lethal doses of radiation may shorten the human life span and increase the occurrence of various forms of cancers particularly leukaemia.

Ionizing radiations are widely used in tumor therapy. The basis for the treatment is the increased frequency of chromosomal breakage and resultant lethality in cells undergoing mitosis compared with cells in interphase. Tumors usually contain more mitotic cells than most normal tissue and so more tumor cells are destroyed than normal cells.

Table 6.A: Types of mutations and their features

Major types of mutations and their distinguishing features

Basis of classification	Major types of mutations	Major features
Origin	Spontaneous	Occurs in absence of known mutagen
	Induced	Occurs in presence of known mutagen
Cell type	Somatic	Occurs in nonreproductive cells
	Germ-line	Occurs in reproductive cells
Expression	Conditional	Expressed only under restrictive conditions (such as high temperature)
	Unconditional	Expressed under permissive conditions as well as restrictive conditions
Effect on function	Loss-of-function (knockout, null)	Eliminates normal function
	Hypomorphic (leaky)	Reduces normal function
	Hypermorphic	Increases normal function
	Gain-of-function (ectopic expression)	Expressed at incorrect time or in inappropriate cell types
Molecular change	Base substitution	One base pair in duplex DNA replaced with a different base pair
	Transition	Pyrimidine (T or C) to pyrimidine, or purine (A or G) to purine
	Transversion	Pyrimidine (T or C) to purine, or purine (A or G) to pyrimidine
	Insertion	One or more extra nucleotides present
	Deletion	One or more missing nucleotides
Effect on translation	Synonymous (silent)	No change in amino acid encoded
	Missense (nonsynonymous)	Change in amino acid encoded
	Nonsense (termination)	Creates translational termination codon (UAA, UAG, or UGA)
	Frameshift	Shifts triplet reading of codons out of correct phase

Because all tumor cells are not in mitosis at the same time irradiation is carried out at regular intervals of several days to enable interphase cells to enter mitosis. Over a period of time most tumor cells are destroyed resulting in hopeful cure. Table 6.A gives details on the type of mutations that occur in DNA bases classified according to their effect.

Mutation Detection in Humans

Humans are obviously not suitable experimental organisms. The techniques developed for the detection of mutations in Drosophila are not suitable to human geneticists. To determine the mutational basis for any human characteristic or disorder, geneticists must first analyse a pedigree that traces the family history as far back as possible. Once any trait has been shown to be inherited, it is possible to predict whether the mutant allele is behaving as a dominant or a recessive and whether it is sex-linked or autosomal.

Dominant mutations are easy to detect. If they are present on the X chromosome, affected fathers pass the phenotypic trait to all their daughters. If dominant mutations are autosomal, approximately 50 percent of the offspring of an affected heterozygous individual are expected to show the trait.

Sex-linked recessive mutations may also be detected by pedigree analysis. The most famous case of a sex-linked mutation in humans is that of **haemophilia**, which was found in the descendants of Queen Victoria. The recessive mutation for haemophilia has occurred since then, many times in human populations the world over.

In a similar manner, it is possible to detect autosomal recessive alleles. Because this type of mutation is "hidden" when heterozygous, it is not unusual for the trait to appear only intermittently through a number of generations. An affected individual and a homozygous normal individual will produce unaffected carrier children. Phenotypic effects manifest differently based on the extent of penetrance (Figure 6.1). Matings between two carriers will produce, on the average, one-fourth affected offspring.

In addition to pedigree analysis, mutation status of the affected individual and their parents can now be easily determined. Human cells are now routinely cultured *in vitro* for any further testing. This procedure has allowed the detection of many more mutations than any other form of analysis. Analysis of enzyme activity, protein migration in electrophoretic fields and direct sequencing of DNA and proteins are among the techniques that have demonstrated wide genetic variation between individuals in human populations. Table 6.B lists mutant loci identified in humans.

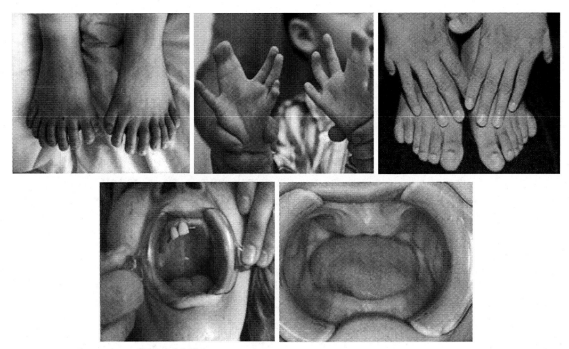

Figure 6.1: Phenotypic effects of different mutations

Table 6.B: Mutant locus identified

a) From biochemical candidates	
Sickle-cell anaemia	
α-thalassaemia	B-globin
β-thalassaemia	α-globin
Haemophilia A	β-globin
Haemophilia B	Factor VIII
Phenylketonuria	Factor IX
Lesch-Nyhan syndrome	Phenylalanine hydroxylase
	Hypoxanthine-guanine
Tay-Sachs disease	phosphoribosyl transferase
Combined immune deficiency	Hexosaminidase A
Adrenal hyperplasia	Adenosine deaminase
Hypercholesterolaemia	Steroid-21 hydroxylase
Hyperlipidaemia	Low-density-lipoprotein (LDL) receptor
*Osteogenesis imperfecta	Apolipoproten CII
*Ehlers-Danlos syndrome	Collagen I
Growth hormone deficiency	Collagen I and collagen III
*Porphyria	Growth hormone
Anti-thrombin III (AT3) deficiency	Uroporphyrinogen decarboxylase AT3
b) From chromosomal mapping	
Chronic granulomatous disease	B-chain of cytochrome b_{-245} (Xp)
Retinoblastoma (RB)	Rb protein (13q)
Duchenne muscular dystrophy	Dystrophin (Xp)
Cystic fibrosis	CF transmembrane conductance regulator (7q)
Familial adenomatous polyposis	APC protein (5q)
Von Recklinghausen neurofibromatosis	NFI protein (17cen)
Wilms tumour	WT protein (11p)
Marfan syndrome+	Fibrillin (15q)
Retinitis pigmentosa (autosomal)	Rhodopsin (3q)
II Mutant locus located	
a) X-chromosome	
Retinitis pigmentosa	Xp
Hypophosphataemia (dominant)	Xp
Choroideraemia	Xq
Emery-Driefuss muscular dystrophy	Xq
Hunter syndrome	Xq

b) Autosomes	
von Hippel-Lindau disease	3p
Huntington chorea	4p
*Familial Alzheimer disease	21q

*Not all cases due to mutations at this locus. †Biochemical candidates located by chromosomal mapping.

As stated earlier, chromosomal aberrations also constitute important category of mutations. Accordingly, the various chromosome abnormalities whether autosomal or X chromosome (addition or deletion) are summarised in Table 6.C whereas microdeletion syndrome of chromosome leading to various clinical presentations are shown in Table 6.D.

Table 6.C. Types of Chromosome Abnormalities

Chromosome Abnormality	Resultant Aberration	Presentation
Triploidy	Three copies of all chromosomes	Usually results in miscarriage
Monosomy		
Autosomal	Single copy of one autosome	Lethal in early pregnancy
X chromosome	Single sex chromosome	Usually lethal during pregnancy, may present during infancy, childhood, or adolescence
Trisomy		
Autosomal	Three copies of an autosome	Lethal during gestation for all autosomes except 13, 18 and 21, which present at birth
Sex chromosome	Extra sex chromosome	Usually identified in late childhood or adulthood
Deletion		
Autosomal	Partial monosomy of one autosome	Usually presents at birth or during early childhood
X chromosome	Partial monosomy of an X chromosome	Variable presentation from birth to adulthood
Duplication		
Autosomal	Partial trisomy	Presents from birth to early childhood

Table 6.D. Recognizable Microdeletion Syndromes Detectable by Fluorescence In Situ Hybridization (Fish)

Syndrome	Deletion	Clinical Description
Prader-Willi	15q12	Hypotonia, obesity, mental retardation (MR), early feeding problems
Angleman	15q12	Seizures, lack of speech, hand flapping
Velocardiofacial	22q11.2	Narrow face, cleft palate, cardiac anomalies
Miller-Dieker	17p13.3	Lissencephaly, wrinkled brow, early death
Williams	7q11.2	Prominent lips, cardiac defects, friendly behavior, MR
Wolf-Hirschhorn	4p16.3	Severe MR, prominent nose.

MOLECULAR BASIS OF MUTATIONS IN HUMANS

If the gene is considered as a linear sequence of nucleotide pairs, following the triplet colour concept, each sequence of three nucleotides specifies a single amino acid in the corresponding polypeptide. Any change/mutation disrupts the coded information. A single change can alter the meaning of the sentence THE CAT SAW THE RAT. Any change, deletion or addition creates various levels of missense.

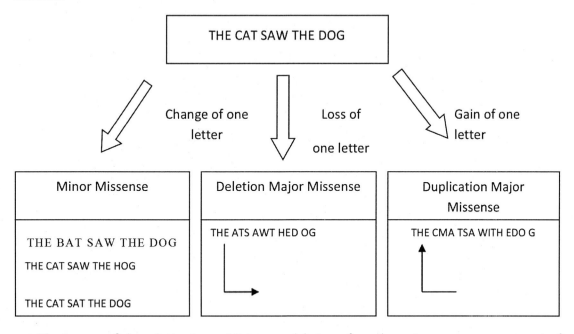

The impact of the substitution, addition, or deletion of one letter in a sentence composed of three-letter words, creating various levels of missense.

The above examples are analogous to base substitutions or point mutations and are used to describe nucleotide substitutions. If a pyrimidine replaces pyrimidine or vice versa a transition results.

If a purine and a pyrimidine are interchanged a transversion results. Further, frameshift mutations may result from the deletion or duplication resulting in garbled message as shown in the above figure.

The diagram below (Figure 6.2) summarises the molecular basis of stable mutations resulting in 12 substitutions. The best example of point mutation is substitution of GAG (glutamic acid) to GUG (Valine) in the opposite strand causing sickle cell anaemia.

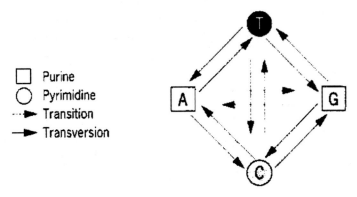

Figure 6.2: Mutational changes due to base substitution

As pointed out earlier, the genetic code is triplet. Diseases due to triplet repeat expansion (dynamic unstable mutations) are common in humans (Table 6.E). The data on how sequence variations cause numerous mutations resulting in various diseases are shown in Figure 6.3. For instance, studies in muscular myopathies including myotonic dystrophy showed that an expansion in the CTG repeats was responsible for the condition (Vasavi et al, 2012).

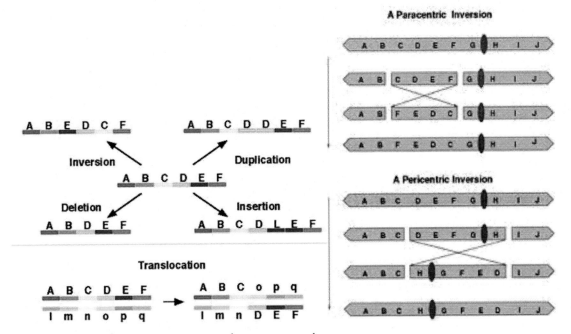

Figure 6.3: Types of sequence variations in chromosomes and gene structure

Table 6.E: Disease Due to Triplet Repeat Expansion

Disease	Sequence Repeat	Number Repeat	Number Mutation	Location Repeat
Huntington disease	CAG	9-35	37-100	Coding
Kennedy disease	CAG	17-24	40-55	Coding
Spino-cerebellar ataxia 1 (SCA 1)	CAG	19-36	43-81	Coding
Spino-cerebellar ataxia 2 (SCA2)	CAG	15-24	35-39	Coding
Machado-Joseph disease (MJD, SCA3)	CAG	12-36	67->79	Coding
Spino-cerebellar ataxia 6 (SCA6)	CAG	4-16	21-27	Coding
Dentatorubral pallidoluysian atrophy (DRPLA)	CAG	7-23	49->75	Coding
Freidreich's ataxia (FA)	GAA	17-22	200-900	Intronic
Myotonic dystrophy	CTG	5-35	50-4000	3'UTR
Fragile X site A (FRAXA)	CGG	6-54	200->1000	5' UTR
Fragile X site E (FRAXE)	CGG	6-25	>200	?
Fragile X site F (FRAXF)	GCC	6-29	>500	?
Fragile 16 site A (FRA16A)	CCG	16-49	1000-2000	?

TERATOGENESIS/CLINICAL TERATOLOGY

Teratogens are agents that can produce a permanent alteration of structure or function after exposure during embryonic or fetal life directly or indirectly. Clinical teratology deals with the relationship between the anomalies in a child and teratogenic exposure and the risk of anomalies to a pregnant woman or child exposed to a teratogen.

Teratogens act at vulnerable periods of embryogenesis (2 to 10 weeks) and fetal development (4 to 12 weeks). Embryonic development is most sensitive to teratogenic effects, though individual differences in susceptibility to teratogen exist. Teratogenic exposures tend to produce characteristic patterns of multiple anomalies rather than single defects.

Teratogenic factors are thought to be responsible for about 10% of all congenital anomalies. These factors fall into several groups.
1. Maternal metabolic imbalance includes factors intrinsic to the mother that cause alterations of the intrauterine environment of the embryo or fetus.
2. Infectious agents can involve the embryo or fetus transplacentally.
3. Ionizing radiations cause damage and can injure the developing embryo.
4. Environmental agents and occupation chemicals are often of concern to pregnant women.
5. Drugs of abuse may damage the health of mother but also may interfere with the development of the embryo or fetus.
6. Medications early in pregnancy cause congenital anomalies eg. Thalidomide, cytotoxic drugs etc.

CHAPTER 7
Multiple Alleles and Polygenic Inheritance

An organism's genotype or set of alleles, determines its phenotype, or observable features. However, a variety of alleles may interact with one another in different ways to specify the phenotype. Mendel's results were groundbreaking, partly because they contradicted the idea that parental traits were permanently blended in their offspring. In some cases, however, the phenotype of a heterozygous organism can actually be a blend between the phenotypes of its homozygous parents. While in a heterozygous situation, the alleles of one parent can completely dominate over the other allele, which is complete dominance, but most often there is incomplete dominance. Alleles are still inherited according to Mendel's basic rules, even when they show incomplete dominance. The two alleles of each gene have differences between them that produces differences in protein function; no single trait can be attributed to a given allele. So while dominance means that one allele masks the effect of the other allele, codominance is when the effects of both the alleles of the gene are apparent in a trait. The human ABO blood groups are an example of multiple alleles. There are four possible phenotypic blood types for this particular gene: A, B, AB, and O. The letters refer to two specific carbohydrate molecules on the surface of red blood cells. The ABO blood groups are formed by various combinations of three different alleles. These alleles exhibit co-dominance.

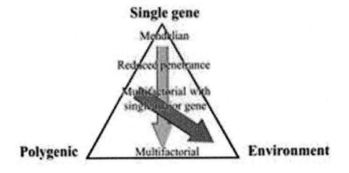

Figure 7.1: Genes and environment

Figure 7.1 describes the influence of environment on single or multiple gene traits where they demonstrate inheritance according to Mendel's laws, nevertheless the environment influences the penetrance and expressivity of the trait. Codominance applies to multiple alleles of a single gene, which is not to be confused with multiple genes that contribute to polygenic inheritance. Polygenic traits are several, for instance the weight or height in humans which depends of multiple genes as well as the environment to an extent (Figure 7.2a). Multiple genes contribute to the inheritance of these traits while being also modified by other factors. These are quantitative characters. In Arachnodactyly, multiple gene mutations may lead to formation of unusually long fingers which is one of the recorded features in patients with Marfan syndrome (Figure 7.2b).

Figure 7.2:

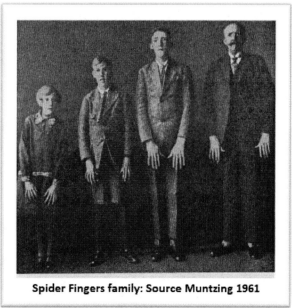

(a)

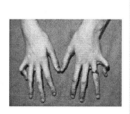

(b) Arachnodactyly in a family due to multigenic inheritance.

8 Patterns of Inheritance

CHAPTER

Because the gene loci are present on both autosomes and sex chromosomes (X & Y) and because of single allelic combination and single-dose effect, four possible inheritance patterns are recognized. Dominant genes require only a single dose while the recessive genes need a double dose. The inheritance patterns are (1) autosomal dominant, (2) autosomal recessive, (3) X-linked dominant and (4) X-linked recessive.

ANALYSIS OF GENETIC DISORDER

Family history of a genetic case:
The first step is to record the family history of the index case/proband. Proband is an affected person who has brought the family to the attention of a clinician. Proband is also called propositus, if male or proposita if female. The procedure starts with gathering information of the disorder, age of onset, duration of complaints and any other major illness. The second step is to collect information regarding the first-degree relatives, i.e. parents, siblings and offsprings of the proband. The following information is recorded-name, surname, date of birth, age, age of death, cause of death and relevant description of the disease (if any). Additionally, the following questions should help in the initiation of a dialogue with the patient or his relatives:
1. Does any relative suffer from similar trait?
   This helps in deciding the pattern of inheritance and subsequently the recurrence risk if any.
2. Does any relative show any other disease which is not present in proband? Cardiac anomalies, ocular malformation or skeletal abnormality in relatives etc. may be asked.
3. Ask for any condition with which any of the relatives has suffered or is suffering.
4. Is the proband an outcome of consanguineous marriage? This may lead to an autosomal recessive trait.
5. What is the ethnic group of the family? Because certain traits are common in some ethnic groups.

The following information may be recorded:
1. Infant deaths, still-births and abortions etc.
2. Illegitimacy should be borne in mind and proper enquiry with the family doctor or medico social worker.
3. Record addresses / contact numbers of relevant family members for follow-up whenever it is required.

The data collected from a family over a number of generations (atleast three) can be represented in a chart using international conventional symbols. Such charts are known as **pedigree charts.**

Disorders caused by a defect in a single gene follow the patterns of inheritance described by Mendel. Individual disorders of this type are often rare but are important because there are over 4000 single gene traits that have been listed. Risks within an affected family are usually high and are calculated by knowing the mode of inheritance and details of the family pedigree. Single gene disorders may be autosomal dominant or recessive.

SINGLE-GENE TRAIT INHERITANCE

Many genetic traits are determined by genes at a single locus; such traits may be dominant or recessive. More than 3000 such conditions, most of which are abnormalities rather than variants of the normal, are known to be single-gene (monogenic diseases/ traits). Table 8.A shows some normal, single gene – dominant and recessive traits in humans.

Table 8. A Single gene traits in human

Dominant traits	Recessive traits
Tongue roller	Non roller
Tongue folder	Non folder
Left thumb on top	Right thumb on top
Widow's peak	No widow's peak
Free Ear lobe	Ear lobe attached
Hair on middle finger digit	Hair absent
Dimple on face	Dimples absent/
Premature grey hair	Normal hair
Absence of a sense of smell	Presence of smell
Right handedness	Left handedness
Normal skin	Albinism

Disease is another aspect of this. A good example is Sickle cell disease which is a group of disorders that affects hemoglobin, the molecule in red blood cells that delivers oxygen to cells throughout the body. The sickle-shaped cells stick to blood vessel walls causing a blockage or slowing down of the flow of blood (Figure 8.1). As a result, oxygen does not reach the tissues giving rise to attacks of sudden, severe pain, called pain crisis. The only cure for SCD is bone marrow or stem cell transplantation. Vast majority of these single gene disorders are of serious nature, none are curable and relatively few are treatable or manageable.

There are over 4000 significant clinical disorders, where the mode of inheritance has been firmly established. These include 750 **autosomal dominant,** 550 **autosomal recessive** and 120 **X-linked disorders.** There are over 447 disorders which show **unifactorial inheritance**.

The patterns followed by single-gene traits within families over a number of generations are determined by the following factors:
1. Whether the trait is dominant or recessive.
2. Whether the gene determining the trait is autosomal or X-linked.
3. Chance distribution of genes from parents to children through the gametes and
4. Factors affecting the expression of a gene, i.e.,
   a. heterogeneity
   b. pleiotropy
   c. reduced penetrance
   d. variable expressivity
   e. variability of age of onset

According to McKusick (1994), over 2000 single gene disorders are known and as on date over 10,000 genes are known to carry various diseases. Broadly speaking, the human genetic diseases are classified as shown in Table 8.B(*i*). Likewise, the prevalence of genetic diseases is summarised in Table 8.B(*ii*). A perusal of the data shows that heritable diseases constitute about 30% of a total of about 40% monogenic disease as per hospital based pediatric practice. The rest accounts for sex-linked and congenital malformations.

Table 8. B(i). Type of Genetic Disease

Single gene	Numerous though individually rare	Autosomal/Sex-linked
(Mendelian)	Clear pattern of inheritance	Dominant and Recessive
	High risk to relatives	
Multifactorial	Common disorders	Drugs and ionising radiations
	No clear pattern of inheritance	
	Low or moderate risk to relatives	
Chromosomal	Mostly rare	Trisomy,
	No clear pattern of inheritance	Monosomy, etc.
	Usually low risk to relatives	
Somatic mutation	Accounts for mosaicism	Cause of neoplasia

Patterns of Inheritance | 81

Table 8.B(ii). Prevalence of Genetic Disease

Type of genetic disease	Estimated prevalence per 1000 population
Single gene	
Autosomal Dominant	2-10
Autosomal recessive	2
X-linked recessive	1-2
Chromosomal abnormalities	6-7
Common disorders with appreciable genetic component	
Congenital malformations	7-10
	20
Total	38-51

Figure 8.1: Sickle cell anemia as a single gene trait (a) Sickling of RBCs (b) Inheritance pattern in Sickle cell disease. (c) Sequence variation in normal adult hemoglobin vs the mutant Hb

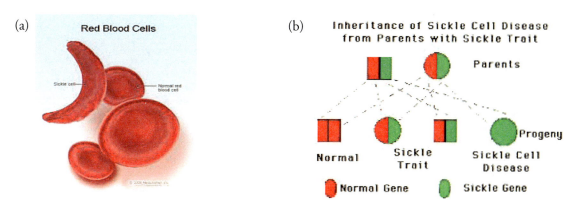

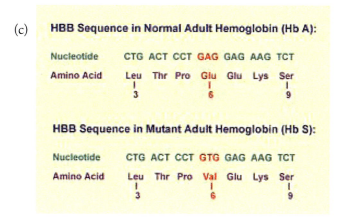

AUTOSOMAL-DOMINANT INHERITANCE

This condition is transmitted vertically from one generation to the next. Males and females are equally affected. When a person has a gene for the condition, the risk of having an affected offspring is 50% for each pregnancy. Genetic risk is always a mathematical estimate of probability governed by chance. Therefore, none, less than half, half, more than half, or all of the offspring could be affected by transmission of autosomal-dominant inheritance.

An individual can carry a gene with a dominant effect without presenting any clinical manifestations. This is called as **lack of penetrance.** The clinical manifestations in autosomal-dominant disorders frequently vary among affected individuals. This is known as variable expressivity. **Penetrance** therefore refers to the number of individuals affected and **expressivity** pertains to the degree to which an individual is affected. These terms are explained earlier.

Criteria for Autosomal Dominant Inheritance
1. Trait should not skip generations (unless penetrance is reduced).
2. An affected person married to a normal person should produce approximately 50% affected offspring (indicating also that the affected individual is heterozygous).
3. Distribution of the trait among sexes should be almost equal.

The severity of many dominant conditions also varies considerably among affected members within a family. The likely severity in any affected offspring is difficult to predict, and a mildly affected parent may have a severely affected child, as in tuberous sclerosis, in which a parent with only skin manifestations of the disorder may have an affected child with infantile spasms and severe mental retardation.

New mutation may account for the presence of a dominant disorder in a person who does not have a family history of the disease. When a disorder arises by a new mutation the risk of recurrence in future pregnancies for the parents of the affected child is negligible. New mutations account for most cases of achondroplasia, a condition that can be easily excluded in the parents. On the other hand, neurofibromatosis may arise by new mutation or be present in mild form in one parent. In dominant conditions an apparently normal parent may occasionally carry a germline mutation; this is associated with a considerable risk of recurrence. A dominant disorder in a person with a negative family history may alternatively indicate non-paternity.

Homozygosity for dominant genes is uncommon, unless two people with the same disorder marry. This may happen preferentially as in achondroplasia. Homozygous achondroplasia is a lethal condition and the risks for offspring are therefore: 25% homozygous affected (lethal); 50% heterozygous affected; 25% homozygous normal. Thus, two out of three living children will be affected.

Diseases due to Autosomal dominant genes

1. Achondroplasia
2. Acute intermittent porphyria
3. Adult polycystic kidney disease
4. Alzheimer's disease (some cases)
5. Epidermolysis bullosa (some forms)
6. Familial hypercholesterolemia
7. Myotonic dystrophy
8. Noonan's syndrome
9. Familial adenomatous polyposis
10. Tuberous sclerosis
11. Malignant hyperthermia
12. Von Hippel-Lindau disease

Autosomal Dominant Traits of Orofacial interest

1. Apert syndrome (with complete penetrance)
2. Axial core defects
3. Amelogenesis imperfecta - I, II & III (with variable expressivity)
4. Anodontia
5. Achondroplasia
6. Acroosteolysis
7. Acrocephalo-syndactyly
8. Coronal dentin dysplasia
9. Cleidocranial dysplasia (with high penetrance variable expressivity)
10. Congenital lip pits
11. Cherubism (with marked penetrance)
12. Chondroectodermal dysplasia
13. Cleft palate and cleft lip or without cleft palate with 80% penetrance
14. Cyclic neutropenia (Gingiva and periodontium)
15. Cronzen syndrome (with complete penetrance)
16. Charcot-Marie-tooth disease 1 A
17. Charcot-Marie-tooth disease 1 B
18. Caffey-Silverman syndrome
19. craniofacial dysostosis with diaphyseal hyperplasia.
20. Dentinogenesis imperfecta, I, II & III
21. Dentatorubral pallidoluysian atrophy
22. Dentin dysplasia I

23. Ehlers-Danlos syndrome
24. Congenital fistulas of the lip
25. Ectodermal Dysplasia
26. Fissured tongue
27. Familial white folded gingivostomatitis
28. Frontometaphyseal dysplasia
29. Larsen syndrome
30. Melnick-Needles syndrome
31. Multiple endocrine neoplasia
32. Maxillary exostosis
33. Mandibular dysostosis (with incomplete penetrance.)
34. Multiple nevoid basal cell carcinoma (with high penetrance, variable expressivity)
35. Multiple Mucosal neuromas
36. Medullary Carcinoma of thyroid.
37. Marfan syndrome (with complete penetrance variable expressivity)
38. Neurofibromatosis
39. Neurofibromatosis of von Recklinghausen
40. Nevoid basal cell carcinoma (with complete, penetrance, variable expressivity)
41. Osteogenesis imperfecta (with variable penetrance and expressivity)
42. Oculodento osseous dysplasia
43. Onycholysis and hypohidrosis
44. Pfeiffer syndrome
45. Polysyndactyly craniofacial syndrome
46. Peutz-Jeghers syndrome (with high penetrance)
47. Pegged or absent Maxillary lateral incisors (with variable expressivity.)
48. Pheochromocytoma (less penetrance)
49. Retinoblastoma
50. Radicular dentin dysplasia
51. Rieger syndrome
52. Saethre-Chotzen syndrome
53. Taurodontism.
54. Treacher Collins syndrome (with high penetrance, variable expressivity)
55. Torus mandibularis (with variable expressivity marked penetrance)
56. Torus platinus (with 100% penetrance)
57. Tricho-dento-osseous syndrome
58. White sponge Nevus (with complete penetrance)

AUTOSOMAL-RECESSIVE INHERITANCE

Criteria for Autosomal Recessive Inheritance
1. Trait often skips generations.
2. There should be an almost equal distribution of affected individuals among sexes.
3. Traits are often found in pedigrees with consanguineous marriages.
4. If both parents are affected, all children should be affected.
5. In most cases of normal people married to affected individuals, all children produced are normal. When at least one child is affected (indicating that the normal parent is heterozygous), then approximately half the children should be affected.
6. Two carriers have a 25% chance of having an unaffected child with two normal genes, 50% chance of having an unaffected child who is a carrier and 25% chance of having an affected child with two recessive genes.

Autosomal recessive disorders are commonly severe. Many of the recognised inborn errors of metabolism follow this type of inheritance. Many complex malformation syndromes are also due to autosomal recessive genes, and their recognition is important in the first affected child in a family because of the 25% risk of recurrence. Prenatal diagnosis for recessive disorders may be possible by performing biochemical assays, DNA analysis, or looking for structural abnormalities in the fetus through amniocentesis.

Autosomal recessive disorders occur in a person whose healthy parents both carry the same recessive gene. The risk of recurrence for future offspring of such parents is 25%. Unlike autosomal dominant disorders there is generally no family history. Although the defective gene may be passed from generation to generation, the disorder generally only appears within a single sibship-that is, within one group of brothers and sisters.

Consanguineous marriages often produce offspring that have rare recessive, and often deleterious, traits. The reason is that through common ancestry (e.g. first cousins have a pair of grandparents in common), an allele found in an ancestor can be inherited on both sides of the pedigree and become homozygous in a child. The occurrence of a trait in a pedigree with common ancestry is often good evidence for an autosomal recessive mode of inheritance. Consanguinity by itself does not guarantee that the trait being examined has an autosomal recessive mode of inheritance; all modes of inheritance are found in consanguineous pedigrees. Conversely, recessive inheritance is not confined to consanguineous pedigrees. Hundreds of recessive traits are known from pedigrees lacking consanguinity.

Diseases due to autosomal recessive genes.
1. Congenital adrenal hyperplasia
2. Deafness (some forms)
3. Diastrophic dwarfism

4. Epidermolysis bullosa (some forms)
5. Friedreich's ataxia
6. Galactosaemia
7. Homocystinuria
8. Hurler's syndrome (Mucopolysaccharidosis I)
9. Laurence-Moon Biedl syndrome
10. Occulocutaneous albinism
11. Phenylketonuria
12. Sickle Cell disease
13. Tay Sachs disease
14. Thalassemia
15. Hemoglobinopathies
16. Gaucher's disease

Autosomal Recessive Traits of Orofacial interest
1. Acrofacial dysostosis
2. Acroosteolysis
3. Acatalasia
4. Amelogenesis imperfecta
5. Chondroectodermal dysplasia
6. Cystic fibrosis
7. Craniodiaphyseal dysplasia
8. Cerebrocostomandibular syndrome
9. Cerebrohepatorenal syndrome
10. Ellis-van Creveld Syndrome
11. Familial osteo dysplasia
12. Hypophosphatasia
13. Mohr syndrome
14. Papillon-Lafevre syndrome
15. Pupal dysplasia
16. Pyknodysostosis
17. Prader-Willi syndrome
18. Progeria
19. Recurrent aphthous ulceration
20. Sclerosteosis
21. Taurodontism
22. Vitamin-D dependent Rickets

A disorder is said to show *genetic heterogeneity* if it can be caused by more than one genetic mechanism. Many such disorders are recognised and counselling can be extremely difficult if the heterogeneity extends to different modes of inheritance. Commonly encountered examples include the various forms of Ehlers-Danlos syndrome, Charcot-Marie-Tooth disease and retinitis pigmentosa, all of which can show autosomal dominant, autosomal recessive and sex-linked recessive inheritance (Table 8.C). Fortunately, progress in molecular genetics is providing solutions to some of these problems. For example, mutations in the gene which codes for rhodopsin, a retinal pigment protein, are found in approximately 50% of families showing autosomal dominant inheritance of Retinitis pigmentosa.

Table 8.C. Hereditary Disorders which can Show Different Patterns Of Inheritance

Disorder	Inheritance patterns
Cerebellar ataxia	AD, AR
Charcot-Marie-Tooth disease (HMSN)	AD, AR, XR
Congenital cataract	AD, AR, XR
Ehlers-Danlos syndrome	AD, AR, XR
Ichthyosis	AD, AR, XR
Microcephaly	AD, AR
Polycystic kidney disease	AD, AR
Retinitis pigmentosa	AD, AR, XR
Sensorineural hearing loss	AD, AR, XR, M

Key: AD = autosomal dominant; AR = autosomal recessive;
XR = sex-linked recessive; M = mitochondrial.

SEX-LINKED INHERITANCE

THE X CHROMOSOME

This medium-size submetacentric chromosome has several genes present on it which have special roles in sex determination. The genes present on the X chromosome are called X-linked or sex-linked. Over 400 X-linked traits have been identified so far on human X chromosome (Figure 8.2).

The X-pter, is homologous to the Y-pter and is called the *pseudoautosomal region*.

Dominant or recessive genes are present on sex chromosomes. Genes carried on the Y chromosomes are referred to as Y-linked. Partially sex-linked genes are those genes which are carried on the homologous portions of the X and Y chromosomes. The overall prevalence of X linked disorders is about 0.5 per thousand.

X-linked inheritance

A male has only one representative of any X-linked gene (always derived from the mother) and hence he is called **hemizygous** rather than **homozygous** or **heterozygous**. Whether recessive or dominant, an X-linked gene is always expressed in the male. A female can be homozygous or heterozygous for any gene.

Since the X chromosome cannot be transmitted from father to son, a male cannot transmit X-linked traits to his male offspring, i.e., father to son. As a father has only one X chromosome which is always transmitted to his daughters, he will always transmit the trait to his daughters in the case of dominant genes or render them carriers in the case of recessive genes.

It may be noted here that though a female has two X chromosomes, only one member of the pair is active; the second one remains condensed and relatively non-functional and is seen as the **Barr body in interphase cells.** Thus, in females, as in males, there is only one functional X, and in heterozygous females, it is a matter of chance whether her paternal or maternal X is in a functional state in a given cell. In heterozygous females, when we refer to X-linked recessive and dominant inheritance, the gene under consideration is functioning only in about half the sex cells.

X-linked recessive inheritance

A classic example is haemophilia. Other examples are listed on page to follow.

Criteria for Sex-linked Recessive Inheritance
1. Most affected individuals are male, heterozygous females are usually unaffected.
2. Affected males result from mothers who are affected or who are known to be carriers (heterozygotes) by having affected brothers, fathers, or maternal uncles.
3. Affected females come from affected fathers and affected or carrier mothers.
4. The sons of affected females must be affected.
5. Approximately half the sons of carrier females should be affected.

The trait is expressed by all males who inherit the gene. Females are affected only if they are homozygous. Thus X-linked recessive diseases are often restricted to males and are uncommon in females.

Mode of Inheritance: In haemophilia, the genotypes are $X_h Y$ for affected male, $X_H X_h$ for carrier female, $X_H X_H$ for normal female and $X_H Y$ for normal male.
1. When an affected male $X_h Y$ marries a normal female $X_H X_H$, all his daughters would be carriers $X_h X_H$ and all his sons would be normal. The carrier daughters will transmit the hemophilia to half their sons.
2. When an affected male $X_h Y$ marries a carrier female $X_h X_H$, half the sons would be affected, half the daughters would be carriers and the other half would be affected. However, this type of combination is rare, since haemophilia in females is severe and may be lethal. Female haemophilic offspring have a good chance of survival with modern therapy.

3. When a carrier female $X_h X_H$ marries a normal male $X_H Y$, half the offspring would be normal, half the sons would be affected, and half the daughters would be carriers.

THE LYON HYPOTHESIS AND X-LINKED-RECESSIVE TRAITS

In Lyon hypothesis, one of the X chromosomes in the female is genetically cancelled at an early stage of embryonal development. This cancellation affects X chromosomes from both maternal and paternal lines. If a female embryo is a carrier of an X-linked-recessive trait, half of the X chromosomes have the normal gene and the other half have the abnormal gene (allele) for the given trait before cancellation occurs. Direct proof of the lyon hypothesis came from identification of the Barr body in normal females as in X chromosome. Genetic evidence also supports the Lyon hypothesis: Females heterozygous for a locus on the X chromosome show a unique pattern of phenotypic expression. Classic haemophilia is a good example which is inherited as an X-linked recessive condition.

In the female carrier, some of the cancelled X chromosomes have the abnormal gene, and others have the normal one. The female carrier is a **mosaic**, that is, she has both normal and abnormal X chromosomes. Because cancellation is random, the number of X chromosomes that remain genetically active and contain the normal or abnormal gene will vary. The female carrier's levels of Factor VIII are often reduced; however, this reduction and the length of coagulation time will vary, depending on the number of X chromosomes that contain the abnormal gene and remain genetically active. Although female carriers of the gene for haemophilia do not have as severe a problem as males, they tend to bleed more than usual after extraction of teeth or scaling and curettage. The variation in the bleeding problem in female carriers of the gene for haemophilia reflects the Lyon hypothesis, as also the X-linked type of amelogenesis imperfecta and hypohidrotic ectodermal dysplasia.

Disease of X linked Recessive Disorders
1. Becker's muscular dystrophy (BMD)
2. Colour blindness
3. Duchenne muscular dystrophy (DMD)
4. Glucose-6-phosphate dehydrogenase deficiency
5. Hunter syndrome
6. Menkes syndrome
7. Mental retardation with or without fragile site
8. Ocular albinism
9. Retinitis pigmentosa

X-linked Recessive Traits of Orofacial interest
1. Amelogenesis imperfecta (snow capped)
2. Anhidrotic ectodermal dysplasia
3. Ectodermal dysplasia
4. Fabry disease (Angio Keratoma)

5. Hemochromatosis
6. Hypohidrotic ectodermal dysplasia
7. Hypomaturation
8. Hypocalcemia
9. Haemophilia-A
10. Haemophilia-B
11. Incontinentia pigmenti
12. Lesch-Nyhan syndrome
13. Norrie disease

Criteria of Sex-Linked Dominant Inheritance
1. The trait does not skip generations.
2. Affected males must come from affected mothers.
3. Approximately half the children of an affected female are affected.
4. Affected females come from affected mothers or fathers.
5. All the daughters, but none of the sons, of an affected father are affected.

X-linked Dominant Inheritance

Examples of X-linked dominant traits are Vitamin D-resistant rickets and Xg blood group. Therefore, X-linked dominant conditions are twice as common in females as in males. The affected male transmits the trait to all his daughters only.

Mode of inheritance
1. When an affected male marries a normal female, he will transmit the trait to all his daughters but to none of his sons.
2. When an affected male marries an affected homozygous female, all the children would be affected, the daughters being homozygous.
3. When an affected male marries an affected heterozygous female, all the daughters and half of the sons would be affected.
4. When a normal male marries an affected homozygous female, all the children would be affected, the daughters becoming heterozygous.
5. When a normal male marries an affected heterozygous female, half the children-sons and daughters-would be heterozygous and affected.

An X-linked dominant gene will give rise to a disorder in both hemizygous males and heterozygous females. The gene is transmitted in families in the same way as X-linked recessive genes, giving rise to an excess of affected females. In some disorders, the condition is lethal in hemizygous males. In this case there will be fewer males than expected in the family, all of whom will be healthy, and an excess of females, half of whom will be affected.

X-Linked Dominant Traits
Rickets - Vitamin D Resistant

X-linked Dominant Traits of Orofacial interest
1. Alport syndrome
2. Fragile X-syndrome
3. Hypophosphatemic Vitamin D resistant rickets
4. Orofaciodigitofacial dysostosis
5. Pseudohypoparathyroidism
6. Incontinentia pigmenti

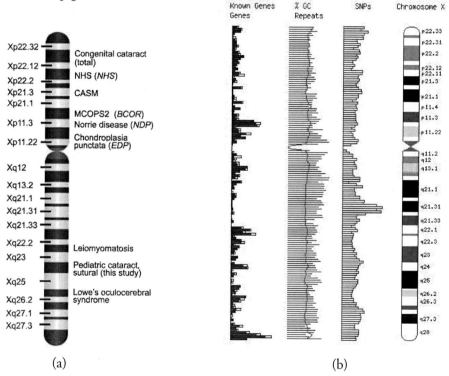

Figure 8.2: (a) Genes of X chromosome related to various disorders

(b) Gene map indicating gene frequency and sequence information on the X chromosome

THE *Y* CHROMOSOME

Y chromosome is a small acrocentric chromosome without any satellite on its short arm. It gives vivid fluorescence with quinacrine stain in metaphase because of a large block of heterochromatin. The Y-pter is homologous to the X-pter and pair with each other during meiosis, and are therefore called the *pseudoautosomal regions*. Close to this, is the region called the testis determining factor (TDF), now said to be located in the sex-determining region of Y chromosome (SRY). Deletion or translocation of SRY gene leads to conditions such as XY females or XX males respectively.

Y-linked Inheritance This is also known as holandric inheritance. The common example is hairy ears (hypertrichosis pinnae auris) in humans, especially males (Figure 8.3). As the Y chromosome is found only in males the non-homologous Y-linked genes are found only in males and are always expressed phenotypically. Males are affected, with transmission being directly from father to the son. This pattern of inheritance has been suggested for such conditions as porcupine skin and webbed toes and these conditions are very rare.

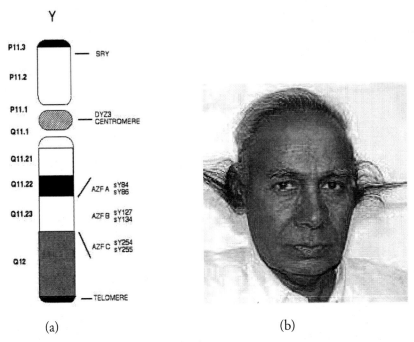

Figure 8.3: (a) Y-chromosome genes related to Y-linked inheritance (b) Auricular hypertrichosis-Y-linked trait

CHAPTER 9
Genetics of Syndromes

Syndrome as defined in Mosby's Dental Dictionary, "is a group of signs and symptoms that occur together and characterize a disease". Hundreds of syndromes have been described in medical specialities. From a genetic point of view, however, two major classes are recognized based on the involvement of sex chromosomes and autosomes. In addition, syndromes associated with cleft lip, cleft palate and tooth, nail or head and neck syndromes are of considerable interest from the orofacial genetics point of view.

VARIATION IN CHROMOSOME NUMBER - AN OVERVIEW

Variation in chromosome number ranges from the addition or loss of one or more chromosomes to the addition of one or more haploid sets of chromosomes. Gains or loses of one or more chromosomes, but not a complete set, is **aneuploidy** as against **euploidy,** where complete haploid sets of chromosomes are found. If there are three or more sets, the term **polyploidy** is applicable. Those with three sets are specifically **triploid.** Table 9. A provides a useful frame-work for the various terms.

Table 9.A. Terminology for Variation In Chromosome Numbers

Term	Explanation
I. Aneuploidy	2n plus or minus chromosomes
Monosomy	2n-1
Trisomy	2n+1
Tetrasomy, pentasomy, etc.	2n+2, 2n+3, etc.
II. Euploidy	Multiples of n
Diploidy	2n
Polyploidy	3n, 4n, 5n, ….
Triploidy	3n
Tetraploidy, pentaploidy, etc.	4n, 5n, etc.
Autopolyploidy	Multiples of the same genome
Allopolyploidy	Multiple of different genomes

CHROMOSOME COMPOSITION AND SEX DETERMINATION IN HUMANS

In the standard system of nomenclature, a normal human chromosome complement is 46,XX for a female and 46,XY for a male. The total chromosome number is given first, followed by the description of the sex chromosomes, and finally, a description of autosomes and any extra sex chromosomes. For example, a male with an extra X chromosome would be 47,XXY. A female with a single X chromosome would be 45,X. Since all the autosomes are numbered, it is customary to describe their changes by referring to their addition (+) or deletion (-). For example, a female with trisomy 21 would be 47,XX,+21.

I: AUTOSOMAL SYNDROMES

(1) Trisomy 13 (Patau Syndrome), 47,XX or XY,+13, and Other Trisomic Disorders

Patau syndrome affects one in twenty thousand live births. Disorder is characterised by multiple abnormalities in various organs. Seventy percent of live-born infants die within the first seven months of life. Diagnostic features are cleft palate, cleft lip, congenital heart defects, polydactyly of hands and feet, and severe mental retardation, anomalies of the external genitals etc. Mortality is very high in the first year of life.

Other autosomal trisomies are known but are extremely rare. These include trisomy 8 (47,XX or XY,+8) and cat's eye syndromes, partial trisomies of an unknown, small acrocentric chromosomes (47,XX or XY, [+acrocentric]).

(2) Trisomy 18 (Edward Syndrome), 47,XX or XY,+18

Edward syndrome affects one in ten thousand live births. Most affected individuals are female, with 80 to 90% mortality by two years of age. The affected usually have a small nose and mouth, a receding lower jaw, abnormal ears, and a lack of distal flexion creases on the fingers. There is limited motion of the distal joints and a characteristic posturing of the fingers in which the little and index fingers overlap the middle two. The syndrome is usually accompanied by severe mental retardation.

(3) Trisomy 21 (Down Syndrome), 47,XX or XY,+21

Down syndrome affects about one in seven hundred live births, is most frequent of the trisomies and is due to non-disjunction. The affected individuals show mild to moderate mental retardation, have congenital hearth defects and a very high (1/100) risk of acute leukaemia. They are usually short and have a broad, short skull, hyperflexibility of joints and excess skin on the back of the neck. The physician John Langdon Down first described this syndrome in 1866. It was the first human syndrome found to be due to a chromosomal disorder, discovered by Jerome Lejeune, a physician in Paris who published this finding in 1959. An interesting aspect of this syndrome is the increased incidence among children of older mothers. The face is characterized by slanted eyes. Patients are generally shorter than normal, heart abnormalities are present in more than 30% of individuals.

The intelligence level varies from near normal to marked retardation. Dentition anomalies, hypodontia in both dentition are seen. Gingival and periodontal disease, dental caries, microdontia is common, enamel hypocalcification is also seen. Premature loss of teeth, especially the mandibular central incisors, caused by alveolar bone loss is frequently seen, and oligodontia (fewer teeth than normal) and abnormally shaped teeth can occur with delayed eruption.

Muriel Davidson of Jackson Laboratory, USA, developed the first mouse model for Down syndrome and stated "Elucidating Down syndrome in a model is a crucial first step towards the development of therapies and interventions for this disorder. For the first time, therapies, treatments and experimental diets that might help DS patients and improve the quality of their lives can be developed and tested".

(4) Cri-du-Chat Syndrome, 46,XX or XY,5p-

The syndrome known as **cri-du-chat** is so called because of the cat-like cry that the affected infants show. Microcephaly, congenital heart disease, and severe mental retardation are also common. This disorder arises from a deletion in short arm of chromosome 5; most other deletions studied (4p-, 13q-, 18p-, 18q-) also result in microcephaly and severe mental retardation. The rarity of viable deletion heterozygotes is consistent with the fact that viable monosomics are rare. An individual heterozygous for a deletion is, in effect, monosomic for that region of the chromosome that is deleted. Evidently, monosomy or heterozygosity for large deleted regions of a chromosome are generally lethal in human beings.

(5) Wolf-Hirschhorn Syndrome

Wolf-Hirschhorn syndrome results from a deletion on the short arm (p) of chromosome 4. Most newborns with the deletion in the short arm of chromosome have a cleft palate and intelligence quotient is less than 30. This affects many parts of the body with delayed growth and development, hypotonia and intellectual disability. The size of the deleted region may vary and larger deletions associate with more severe abnormalities. Most of the cases happen as a result of a random event during the formation of reproductive cells.

II: SEX-CHROMOSOME SYNDROMES

(1) Turner Syndrome 45,X: Patients with Turner syndrome and female phenotype in the majority of cases, have a karyotype with normal 44 autosomes and only one X chromosome. Most cases of Turner syndrome are due to non-disjunction of the X chromosome in the paternal sex cell. Clinically, the females are of short stature with webbed neck and edema of the hands and feet and frequently exhibit a low hairline on the nape of the neck. The chest is broad with wide-spaced nipples. The aorta is frequently abnormal, and body hair is sparse. The external genitals appear infantile, and the ovaries are not developed; therefore, these individuals have primary amenorrhea (abnormal temporary or permanent cessation of the menstrual cycle). Buccal smears from the oral mucosa show absence of Barr bodies.

Karyotypes other than 45,X also lead to Turner phenotype. These include mosaic individuals with two apparent cell lines, the most common chromosome combinations being 45,X/46,XY and 45,X/46,XX. They may also be cases with a partial deletion in the X chromosome. The variability of presentation depends on the degree of mosaicism in these cases. In cases where the pubertal developmental takes place and fertility is retained, mother to daughter transmission of these X deletions is also possible. Turner syndrome is observed in about 1 in 2000 female births, a frequency much lower than that for Klinefelter syndrome. One explanation for this difference is the observation that a substantial majority of 45,X fetuses die *in utero* and are aborted spontaneously.

(2) **47,XXX Syndrome:** The presence of three X chromosomes along with a normal set of autosomes (47,XXX) results from maternal non-disjunction errors during meiosis. Seen in about 1 of 1200 female births and shows highly variable expression. Frequently, 47,XXX women are perfectly normal. In other cases, underdeveloped secondary sex characteristics, sterility, and mental retardation may occur. In rare instances, 48,XXXX and 49,XXXXX karyotypes have been reported. The syndromes associated with these karyotypes are similar to but more pronounced than the 47,XXX. Thus, the presence of additional X chromosomes appears to disrupt the delicate balance of genetic information essential to normal female development. Three or four barr bodies respectively are present in this syndrome.

(3) **Klinefelter Syndrome 47,XXY:** This condition (XXY) occurs when an ovum carrying two X chromosomes is fertilized by a sperm with a Y chromosome. Majority of cases result from non-disjunction of the X chromosome in the ova of older females. Affected individuals are of male phenotype, and the condition often can be detected only after puberty. The patients are taller than normal and have wide hips and a female pubic hair distribution. About 50% have gynecomastia, intelligence levels are lower than normal in 10% of affected individuals. The penis appears normal with smaller and harder testis that lack seminiferous tubules.

The maxilla is slightly hypoplastic. Buccal smears show the presence of one Barr body. Variations of Klinefelter syndrome also occur and are represented by karyotypes containing XXXY or XXXXY. The greater the number of X chromosomes, the more pronounced the clinical manifestations and the lower the level of intelligence. The maxilla becomes increasingly hypoplastic with increasing number of X chromosomes. Buccal smears show 2 and 3 Barr bodies respectively. Klinefelter syndrome occurs in about 2 of every 1000 male births. The karyotypes 48,XXXY, 48,XXYY, 49,XXXXY and 49,XXXYY are similar phenotypically to 47,XXY, though much rarer, but manifestations are often more severe in individuals with a greater number of X chromosomes.

(4) **47,XYY Condition** Another trisomy involving the sex chromosomes involves males with one X and two Y chromosomes in addition to the normal complement of 44 autosomes (47, XYY). It is now known that many XYY males do not exhibit any form of anti-social behaviour and lead normal lives. It can be concluded that there is no direct correlation between the extra Y chromosome and criminal behaviour.

(5) Fragile-X Syndrome: The most common cause of inherited mental retardation is the **fragile-X syndrome.** It is found in about one in every 1,250 males and about one in every 2,000 females. The symptoms include mental retardation, altered speech patterns, large testes in males, and other physical attributes such as high arched palate, prominent lateral palatine ridges, prognathism, long narrow face, large ears and flexible fingers, macroorchidism after puberty. It is called the fragile-X syndrome because it is related to a region at the tip of the X chromosome that breaks more frequently than other chromosomal regions. However, the break is not required for the syndrome, and the fragile-X chromosome is usually identified by the lack of chromatin condensation at the site. The gene responsible for the syndrome is called *FMR-1*, for fragile-X mental retardation-1 which has a DNA segment of CGG triplet that is repeated abnormally (>200 times), thus silencing the gene. Loss of protein affects the nervous system and produces all other signs and symptoms of disease.

An interesting property of the syndrome is that approximately 20% of males with the fragile-X chromosome do not have symptoms but have grandchildren that do have the symptoms (have dynamic mutations in the triplet repeat sequences). The daughters of the symptomatic males also lack symptoms.

III: CLEFT-LIP AND CLEFT-PALATE SYNDROMES

Syndromes of cleft lip and cleft palate are the single most common defects affecting the oro-facial structures in man and studied in considerable detail. In general, such syndromes cause extreme disfiguring and affect function to a considerable extent. Genetic factors play a key role in the etiology. Several excellent reviews on the subject are available (see Ross and Johnson, 1972, Kernahan 1968, Gorlin et. al, 1990) in respect of syndromes of cleft lip, clefts of primary and secondary palate and rarely clefts of the facial skeleton such as clefts and mandibular clefts. Of the 100 syndromes described by Gorlin et. al. (1990), about 30% are the result of single gene mutations. Based upon embryology, eight categories of such syndromes have been recognised as listed below:-

1. Unilateral incomplete cleft of the primary palate.
2. Complete cleft of the primary palate, ending at the incisive foramen.
3. Bilateral complete cleft of the primary palate.
4. Incomplete isolated cleft of the secondary palate.
5. Complete cleft of the primary soft and hard palate.
6. Unilateral complete cleft of the primary and secondary palates.
7. Bilateral complete cleft of the primary and secondary palates.
8. Incomplete cleft of the primary palate and incomplete cleft of the secondary palate.

In table 9.B, a summary of syndromes of cleft lip and palate is presented. Most of the syndromes of CL(P)/CP are of genetic origin, and follow autosomal dominant inheritance, though Larsen syndrome and Diastrophic dwarfism follow autosomal recessive pattern. Cleft palate syndromes viz. oto-palato-digital syndromes are X-linked.

Table 9.B. Syndromes Associated with Clefts of the Lip and/or Palate

Syndromes	Inheritance pattern	CL (P) or CP	Frequency of Clefts
Genetic			
Lip-pit	A.D.	CL(P)	30 per cent
Larsen's	A.R.	CP	Nearly 100 per cent
Ocular hypertelorism of Grieg	A.D.	CL(P)	Frequent
Cleidocranial dysostosis	A.D.	CP	Submucous or CP frequent
Craniofacial dysostosis	A.D.	CP	High arch or CP frequent
Diastrophic dwarfism	A.R.	CP	25 per cent
Mandibulofacial dysostosis	A.D.	CP	High frequency
Oto-palato-digital	X-linked	CP	High frequency
Chondrodystrophia calcificans congenita	?	CP	25 per cent
Cornelia de Lange	?	CP	10 per cent
Smith-Lemli-Opitz	?	CP	40 per cent
Nongenetic			
Arthromyodysplasia congenita	-	CL(P)	Rare
Trisomy 13-15	-	CL(P)	Occasionally
Trisomy 17-18	-	CL(P)	Nearly 100 per cent
XXY, XXXY	-	CL(P)	50 per cent
Moebius syndrome	-	CL(P)	5 to 7 per cent
Oculoauriculovertebral dysplasia	-	CL(P)	Occasionally
Congenital rubella	-	CL(P)	Common
Thalidomide	-	CL(P)	Common

ad = autosomal dominant, ar = autosomal recessive.
cp = cleft palate, cl(p) = cleft lip with or without cleft palate.
(reproduced from Poole (1975): genetics of cleft-lip and palate)

As of now the inheritance of these syndromes is controversial. Simple mendelian inheritance is suggested for some while the involvement of individual chromosomes is implicated in others. Molecular genetic studies of CP ± CL in Iceland has indicated involvement of a gene on X chromosome hence sex-linked inheritance.

Isolated cleft palate and cleft lip with or without palate is said to be polygenic. According to Kingston (1997), the risk of recurrence in siblings for cleft lip and palate is 4% while for cleft palate alone the risk is much less (2%). Sex-wise distribution and incidence in world population has been reviewed by Poole (1975) and Morgan (1993). According to Verma (1995), CL/CP congenital malformations in India constitute 1-3 per 1000 as per the national multi-centre study.

Kumar et. al. (1998) have studied the incidence of cleft lip and palate in Manipal for the period 1988 – 1991. The risk of every parent having a child with a cleft is 1 in 700. The recurrence risk for first degree relatives is about 3.3% for CL/P and for isolated CP it is 2%. Once parents have a child with a cleft, the risk after two affected children rises to 9-12%. So, parents and young adults should be counseled by a geneticist so that they are in a better position to make decisions about future pregnancies. The findings from their work are similar to that of Reddy (1983) for a similar study from Mangalore.

IV. TOOTH AND NAIL SYNDROMES

Syndromes involving tooth and nail and other characteristics are relatively rare and the published data is scanty. Ectodermal and chondroectodermal dysplasia are rare. Hereditary disease associated with tooth abnormalities is sparse, with scant eyebrows, eye lashes, brittle, poorly formed nails and reduced sweating, which can be an autosomal dominant or recessive genetic trait.

Review of literature of traits together with related characters is presented below:

1.	Ectodermal dysplasia (Autosomal dominant)	..	Giansanti et. al. (1974)
		..	Freire- Maia and Pinheiro (1984)
2.	Hypoplastic enamel, Onycholysis and hypohidrosis (Autosomal dominant)	..	Witkop et. al. (1975)
3.	Hypodontia, nail dysgenesis, (Holandric?)	..	Hudson and Witkop (1975)
4.	Trichodentoosseous syndrome (Autosomal Dominant) (kinky hairs, thick cornified nails and microdontia)	..	Batayneh, O (2012)
5.	Tooth and Nail syndrome (Autosomal dominant)	..	Akyuz and Atasu (1993)
6.	Anodontia -	..	Scherer et al (1990)
	–Partial anodontia	..	Ekstrand and Thomsson (1988)
	–Multiple anodontia	..	Bondarets (1990)
7.	Chondroecto dermal dysplasia (Autosomal dominant)	..	Prabhu et al (1992).

Akyuz and Atasu (1993) reported a case of a 5 ½ year old patient from Istanbul, Turkey with the following features. This appears to be the best described syndrome under this category.

1. Left and right first maxillary, primary molars absent
2. Maxillary right, lateral incisor-missing
3. Anterior teeth small, sharp and cone shaped.
4. Maxillary, central teeth hypoplastic.
5. Lower chin prognathic.
6. Germ in permanent teeth absent in panoramic radiograph.
7. Eye brows sparse.
8. Nails poorly developed, brittle.

The authors have studied the pedigree of the patient and concluded the inheritance to be autosomal dominant (rarely recessive). The study was supplemented with dermatoglyphic studies involving palmar and plantar configurations and total finger ridge count of the entire family. Further association studies between features like periodontitis and coronary artery disease was also suggested by research work (Madhavi et al, 2019).

Orofacial Syndromes (Head and Neck) Sedano (see Ibsen and Phelaus Oral Pathology) has classified the syndromes under the following categories.

I. INHERITED DISORDERS AFFECTING THE GINGIVA AND PERIODONTIUM
1. Cyclic Neutropenia
2. Gingival Fibromatosis
3. Laband syndrome
4. Gingival Fibromatosis with hypertrichosis, epilepsy and mental retardation.
5. Gingival fibromatosis with multiple hyaline fibromas.

II. INHERITED DISORDERS AFFECTING THE JAW BONES AND FACIES
1. Cherubism
2. Chondroectodermal dysplasia
3. Cleidocranial dysplasia
4. Gardner syndrome
5. Mandibulofacial dysotosis
6. Multiple Nevoid basal cell carcinoma syndrome and gorlin syndrome
7. Osteogenesis imperfecta
8. Torus mandibularis
9. Torus palatinus
10. Maxillary exostosis

III. INHERITED DISORDERS AFFECTING THE ORAL MUCOSA
1. Isolated clept palate and cleft lip with or without cleft palate (Multifactorial)
2. Hereditary hemorrhagic telangiectasia
3. Multiple mucosal neuromas, Medullary carcinoma of the thyroid gland and Phaeochromocytoma
4. Peutz-Jeghers syndrome
5. White sponge Nervus

IV. INHERITED DISORDERS AFFECTING THE TEETH
1. Amelogenesis Imperfecta
2. Dentinogenesis Imperfecta
3. Dentin Dysplasia
4. Hypohidrotic ectodermal Dysplasia (X linked recessive)
5. Hypophosphatasia

6. Hypophasphatemic Vitamin D resistant Rickets
7. Pegged or absent maxillary lateral incisors
8. Taurodontism

Crespi (see Regezi and Seiubba's Oral pathology) has discussed the various syndromes under two categories.

1. METABOLIC DISORDERS and GENETIC ABNORMALITIES.

Syndromes of interest to the dentist can be categorized by the stage of development in which they become clinically identifiable, either soon after birth or later in life. Syndromes that are identifiable soon after birth result from either genetic defects or adverse influences by a clinically obvious feature, within one of the following groups;

a. Deficient mandibular development
b. Deficient maxillary development
c. Defective skin formation or discoloration of skin

Syndromes that become apparent later in life can be either genetically determined or acquired by various other pathologic mechanisms such as autoimmune conditions, degenerative diseases, or infections. Several examples of late onset syndromes of genetic origin are characterized by the development of multiple hamartomatous or neoplastic enlargements, while others are manifest by unusual inflammatory lesions. Many acquired syndromes consist of multiple clinical findings that are diverse pathophysiologic consequences of an underlying abnormality such as anaemia.

2. DEVELOPMENTAL SYNDROMES

Developmental syndromes with oral features present a diagnostic challenge because most examples occur relatively rarely which limits the clinicians opportunity to gain direct familiarity with many examples. Also, the diverse manifestations that characterize many syndromes can become confused with the coincidental occurrence of several abnormalities caused by unrelated conditions. The diagnosis of patients with multiple abnormalities requires correlation of the pattern of observed abnormalities with features of recognized syndromes. This frequently involves anatomic and functional abnormalities not directly related to oral structures.

CHAPTER 10
Rare and Severe Genetic Disorders

There are several such disorders but just to give the reader a flavour of some known ones, please read below:

Hypertrichosis: People with hypertrichosis have excessive hair on the shoulders, face, and ears. Studies have implicated it to a rearrangement involving a paracentric inversion mutation of band q22 of chromosome 8. The mutation could be spontaneous in nature. It may be congenital or acquired.

Red Hair: Having red hair is a genetic mutation. Hair color is made up of two main pigments. Eumelanin is the more common pigment and is responsible for all hair colors other than red. The other pigment, pheomelanin is less common and is responsible for red hair and the orangish red look. With MC1R doing its job properly, it turns pheomelanin into eumelanin. With a disruption of the MC1R gene, the protein cannot work properly and a build of pheomelanin occurs. Other common traits that are associated with people with the red hair gene include very fair skin and more sensitivity to ultraviolet radiation, meaning they can sunburn easily. Individual hair strands are thicker than those of people with other hair colors, but they have up to 30% strands. This means balding and thinning can be a problem.

Freckles*:* This is actually related to red hair in a way. Freckles can result from time spent in the sun, but some are because of genetic causes. Skin cells called melanocytes react to sunlight and increase the production of melanosomes to protect against the sun's UV rays thus changing the colour of outer skin cells called keratinocytes. In most people, these melanocytes are spread out fairly evenly, but in some cases, especially in people with red hair, the cells tend to clump together. As with red hair, it is the MC1R proteins that are the main issue. A substitution error on the MC1R gene leads to errors in instructions for making the MC1R protein. When sunlight strikes the clumps, the orangish-red freckles start popping out.

Blue eyes: It well known fact that having blue eyes is a genetic mutation! About 6,000 to 10,000 years ago a rare genetic mutation occurred that resulted in a person having blue eyes. This one individual has now become a common ancestor to all people with blue eyes according to researchers. The gene involved is the OCA2 gene. The OCA2 gene codes for the P protein, which is involved in the production of melanin. By switching off the gene, the production of melanin in the iris is reduced and turns brown eyes to blue.

Attached or free earlobes- *Just take some time just long enough to look at your ear lobes.* This is also a genetic mutation and some people have attached while some have free ones. Meta-analysis studies show a polygenic association with the structure of the ear lobe which has been a matter of debate since the early 20th century.

Progeria: This genetic disorder is as rare as well as severe. The classic form of the disease, called Hutchinson-Gilford Progeria, causes accelerated aging. The disease is caused by a mutation in the LMNA gene, a protein that provides support to the cell nucleus. Other symptoms of progeria include rigid (sclerotic) skin, full body baldness (alopecia), bone abnormalities, growth impairment, and a characteristic "sculptured" nasal tip.

11

CHAPTER

Developmental Genetics

This is the branch of genetics concerned with the role of genes in orchestrating the changes/processes that occur during development right from the fetal stage through adulthood. Currently this is one of the hottest fields in molecular biology.

Much of our understanding of the genetic mechanisms that guide human embryonic development depends on studies carried out in model organisms such as fruitflies (*Drosophila melanogaster*), worm (*Caenorhabitis elegans*), frog (*Xenopus*) and even plants (*Arabidopsis thaliana*) because of the powerful genetic and embryological experimental methods conducted on them. The results from those studies were then extrapolated to the understanding of the human biology because many cellular and molecular mechanisms operating during human development are similar to those used during the development of invertebrate organisms. Mammalian model organisms such as mice and rats are also useful because the actual tissue interactions and movements are conserved; development of heart, brain, lungs, liver in mouse embryos show much similarity with human embryos. Model organism studies not only have provided tools for understanding human development but also served as a platform for the development of new therapies relevant to organ transplantation and regeneration. In the foregoing, a brief account of how the genes govern some developmental processes, has been discussed.

Fertilization: determination, differentiation, cell to cell interaction

For sexual reproduction, successful fertilization for producing offsprings is a necessary process. Fertilization takes place by union of a set of haploid chromosomes from ovum and sperm (gametes) to produce a diploid zygote. The formation of zygote from gametes requires a series of well-coordinated events including gamete activation, recognition, signaling, adhesion and fusion (Primakoff and Myles, 2002; Singson et al. 2001). Genetic analysis of fertilization products can be done by describing unique gamete characteristics defined by advanced techniques like genome sequencing, linkage maps and targeted gene sequencing methods. These have paved way for genetic analysis of various species.

Advancement in reproductive genetics, a sub-field of medical genetics involved in conducting different tests for predicting possible outcomes of future pregnancies has led to novel ideas including the realization of gene therapeutic modalities. This is achieved by analyzing genetic material like chromosomes, genes, DNA, RNA and gene products for accessing genetic changes that have likelihood of causing some disease during/after pregnancy in the offspring.

In mammalian fertilization, sperm mitochondria are incorporated into the oocyte, specific mitochondrial proteins are ubiquinated in the spermatid. Sperm mitochondria are destroyed in the oocyte by ubiquitin-stimulated proteolysis. Only maternal mitochondria are inherited by the zygote. Mitochondrial genome is also of importance with respect to disease and maternal inheritance.

The present knowledge and best model for studying fertilization is by conducting research in marine invertebrates and vertebrate model systems; *C. elegans* has emerged as powerful system. Common genetic model systems like Yeast, *Chlamydomonas*, *Caenorhabditis Elegans*, *Drosophila*, Zebrafish (*Danio Rerio*) and mouse have also contributed to the growth spurt in the area of clinical genetic research.

Cell division: Cell division occurs to replicate cells by mitosis and meiosis. In mitosis the body cells replicate to form two cells with identical genetic makeup. Whereas, meiosis occurs in germ cells, the genetic component is divided and there is a decrease in the chromosomal number by half, to produce gametes (Ovum and sperms). Germ cells contain 23 (single set) chromosomes, half of the genetic material of normal somatic cells. When the haploid ovum and sperm unite, they form the zygote which is diploid, with human chromosome complement of 46 chromosomes or 23 pairs.

Gametogenesis: Spermatogenesis in males produces four mature sperms, whereas Oogenesis in the female produces one mature ovum.

Conception: It is defined as the union of a single egg and sperm and marks the beginning of a pregnancy.

Fertilization: Fertilization is an essential biological process in sexual reproduction and comprises a series of molecular interactions between the sperm and egg. It takes place in the outer third portion of the uterine tube. When sperm successfully penetrates the membrane surrounding the ovum, both sperm and ovum are enclosed within the membrane and the membrane become impenetrable to other sperms, called zona reaction.

After formation of zygote mitotic cellular replication begins as the zygote travels the length of the uterine tube into the uterus. This voyage takes place in 3-4 days. Fertilized egg divides rapidly without increase in size, successive smaller cells called blastomeres are formed with each division. Within three days morula, a solid ball of 16 cells is formed and it is still surrounded by protective zona pellucida. The blastomeres are separated into two parts; the trophoblast which gives rise to placenta and the embryoblast, which give rise to embryo.

Genetic approaches have been informative and focusing on the roles of secreted and cell surface proteins, expressed in a sex-specific manner, that mediate sperm-egg interactions in mammalian fertilization. It is important to know how the sperm interaction with the female reproductive tract, zona pellucida, and the oolemma have aided interventions and artificial reproductive techniques. Progress has been made in elucidating the mechanisms that reduce polyspermy and ensure that eggs normally fuse with only a single sperm.

Fertilization takes place in a two-step process/mechanism. Sperm Izumo1, a binding protein on the surface of the sperm, recognizes its receptor Juno (a part of the family of folate receptor proteins), on the egg surface and this is followed by fusion of two plasma membranes (Bianchi et al., 2014). Human Izumo1 forms a high-affinity complex with Juno and undergoes a major conformational change within its N-terminal domain upon binding to the egg-surface receptor. The understanding of the molecular basis of sperm-egg recognition, cross-species fertilization, and barrier to polyspermy thus promises benefits for the development of newer non-hormonal birth control methods and fertility treatments for humans and other species of mammals.

Implantation:

Between 6 to 10 days, the zona pellucida degenerates and trophoblast attaches to uterine endometrium of the fundal region. The trophoblast secretes enzymes that enable it to burrow into endometrium until the entire blastocyst is covered in a process called implantation. Chronic villi or finger like projections develop from trophoblast and extend into the blood-filled spaces of endometrium for obtaining oxygen and nutrients from the maternal blood stream. After implantation the endometrium is called deciduas and the portion under the blastocyst where chorionic villi taps into the maternal blood vessels is called deciduas basalis. The portion covering the blastocyst is the deciduas capsularis and the portion lining the rest of the uterus is the deciduas vera. During a certain window period, the normally hostile endometrium turns favourable to the embryo for allowing implantation. The Wnt5a gene along with its co-receptors Ror1 and Ror2 is important in directing the embryo to getting implanted in the womb.

Important development-regulating genes

Not all genes are involved in the function of developmental control - some genes are required in all cells (housekeepers), while others have specialized functions and are only required in certain differentiated cell types (effector genes). Developmental control genes have a defined mutant phenotype, and their structure, function and identity have been remarkably consistent across various model organisms. Homeotic genes (Hox) encode a family of transcriptional regulators, function in governing the developmental fate of a particular region of the body. The homeobox (HOX), a 180-base pair consensus sequence is found in homeotic genes. Homeodomain is the protein domain encoded by the homebox and promotes the binding of the protein to the DNA. The presence of this *master switch gene*, regulates the development of whole groups of other genes. Their genomic organisation and molecular regulation is highly complex where they presumably act as binary switches and define whether the development goes on in one direction or another.

The Hox genes were discovered in Drosophila (Bridges and Morgan, 1923), where they exist in two separate gene clusters: the Antennapedia and Bithorax complexes (ANT-C and BX-C, respectively). Clustering is an intrinsic property of Hox genes that is indispensable for proper regulation of Hox gene expression. Hox gene expression within the cluster correlates with the distribution of histone modifications associated with inactive (trimethylation at Lys27 of histone H3, H3K27m3) and active (trimethylation at Lys4 of histone H3, H3K4m3) chromatin throughout the Hox cluster (Schuettengruber et al., 2007).

Hox gene mutants are interesting mutants in which one cell type follows the developmental pathway normally followed by other cell types. For example, mutations in HoxD13 in humans can cause a genetic condition called synpolydactyly, in which people are born with extra fingers or toes that may also be fused together. The Hox cluster is a good example of how developmental genes can be both preserved and modified through evolution and how a transcription factor can target genes to switch 'on or off' to activate a particular genetic program.

There is a rich prevalence of transcription factors and signaling molecules among developmental control genes. Many of these transcription factors are both necessary and sufficient to initiate specific developmental programs. Dynamic regulation is expected since the genes have to act locally in order to affect specific developmental processes. Regulation occurs at all levels, from the transcriptional to the post-translational level. Understanding of these mechanisms can help achieve targeting of these pathways by designing specific drugs by suitable pharmaceutical programs to make a difference in the dysregulation (during development) leading to human disease.

12 Genetics of Cancer

CHAPTER

Cancer is an informal term for diseases marked by abnormal (mutant) cell proliferation and migration of these rogue cells. Control of normal cell development is lost and cells proliferate inappropriately to form tumours (neoplasms). Neoplasms may be either benign or malignant depending on their ability to metastasize. It is related to environmental mutagens, somatic mutations or maybe a genetic predisposition.

Cancers are divided into four major groups depending on the type of cells originally involved. Most cancers are clonal i.e. arise from a single aberrant cell that clonally proliferates. Currently, there are two theories regarding the cause of cancer, the mutation theory which states that most cancers are due to genetic mutation while viral theory states that most cancers are of viral origin. Both the theories are presently unified.

The genetic basis of both sporadic and inherited cancers has been confirmed by molecular studies. The three main classes of genes known to predispose to malignancy are oncogenes, tumour suppressor genes, and genes involved in DNA repair. In addition, specific mutagenic defects due to environmental carcinogens and viral infections (notably hepatitis B and human papilloma virus) are being identified. Oncogenes are normal genes that when altered or overexpressed, may initiate or promote neoplasia. Oncogenes are conserved in evolution and any alterations cause malignant transformation of normal cells. They were first recognised as viral oncogenes (v-onc) carried by RNA viruses. Sequences homologous to those of viral oncogenes were subsequently detected in the human genome and called cellular oncogenes (c-onc). More than 100 proto-oncogenes have been described and their normal function is for the control of growth and differentiation. Almost all the autosomes harbour proto-oncogenes as shown in table 12.A.

Table 12.A. Chromosomal Localisation Of Proto-Oncogenes In Human Genome

Chromosome No.	Site	Gene
1	q12ter	c-src-2
1	Cen-p21	N-ras
1	p32	Hum Blym^{-1}
3	NA	c-ski
5	q34	c-fms
6	q22-q24	c-myb
7	pter –q22	c-erbB
8	q22	c-mos
8	q24	c-myc
9	q34	c-abl
11	p14.1	C-ras^H
11	q23 –q24	c-ets
12	p12.5-ter	c-ras^K
14	q21 –q31	c-fos
15	q24 –q25	c-fes
17	q21 –q22	c-erbA
20	p34 –p36	c-src-1
22	q11-ter	c-sis

Mutation in a proto-oncogene results in altered, enhanced or inappropriate expression of the gene product leading to neoplasia. Oncogenes act in a dominant fashion in tumour cells in that, a given mutation in one copy of the gene is sufficient to cause neoplasia. Proto-oncogenes may be activated by point mutations, gene amplification or specific chromosomal translocations. Most proto-oncogenic mutations occur at a somatic level, causing sporadic cancers. The mechanism or pathways by which oncogenes and tumour suppressor genes act / interact is not completely clear. However, tumour suppressor genes normally act to control cell proliferation, and loss or inactivation is associated with tumorigenesis. At the cellular level these genes act in a recessive fashion, as loss of activity of both copies of an autosomal gene is required for malignancy to develop. Tumour suppressor gene inactivation occurs in both sporadic and hereditary cancers. Table 12.B lists out some of the neoplasm that are almost always connected with a specific chromosomal abnormality thus making them a diagnostic and prognostic marker in these patients.

Table 12.B. Neoplasms with a Known Chromosomal Defect

Disease	Chromosomal Defect	Breakpoints/ Deletion
1) **Leukaemias (Bone marrow)**		
Chronic myelogenous leukaemia	t(9;22)	9q34.1 and 22q11.21
Acute myeloid leukaemia	t(9;22)	9q34.1 and 22q11.21
	t(8;21)	8q22 and 21q22
Chronic lymphocytic leukaemia	+12	
	t(11;14)	11q13 and 14q32
Acute lymphocytic leukaemia	t(9;22)	9q34.1 and 22q 11.21
	t(12;21)	12p12 and 21q22
2) **Lymphomas (Lymph nodes)**		
Burkitts	t(8;14)	8q24.13 and 14q32.33
Follicular	t(14;18)	14q32 and 18q21
3) **Carcinomas (epithelial tissues of glands)** 85% cancers		
Neuroblastoma, disseminated	del1p	1p31p36
Small cell lung carcinoma	del3p	3p14p23
Papillary cystadenocarcinoma of ovary	t(6;14)	6q21 and 14q24
Constitutional retinoblastoma	del13q	13q14.13
Wilm's tumor	del11p	11p13
4) **Sarcomas** (embryological mesoderms of bone)	t(X;18)	Xq11.2 and 18q11.2

The symbols are those conventionally used in human cytogenetics are as follows:

1. The long arm of a chromosome is symbolised as q, the short arm as p. For example, 11p refers to the short arm of chromosome 11.
2. A (+) or (–) sign preceding a symbol denotes an extra copy (or a missing copy) of the entire designated chromosome. For example, +6 means the presence of an extra chromosome 6.
3. A (+) or (–) sign following a symbol denotes extra material (or missing material) corresponding to part of the designated chromosomal arm. For example, 11p – refers to a deletion of part of the short arm of chromosome 11.
4. The symbol "t" refers to a translocation. Thus, t(9;22) refers to reciprocal translocation between chromosome 9 and chromosome 22, the derivative philadelphia chromosome is associated with chronic myelogenous leukaemia.

Genetic Basis

A summary of the genetic bases of cancer apart from the chromosome abnormalities is discussed below. Mendelian condition with strong pre-disposition to neoplasia

1. **Syndromes of multiple benign or malignant neoplasia (Autosomal dominant)**

    e.g.
    - Neurofibromatosis
    - Multiple endocrine neoplasia
    - Familial adenomatous polyposis of colon
    - Li Fraumeni syndrome

2. **Abnormalities of DNA repair**

    i. Syndromes associated with other phenotypic abnormality (Autosomal recessive)

    e.g.
    1. Xeroderma pigmentosum
    2. Fanconi anemia
    3. Ataxia telangiectosia

    ii. Hereditary non-polyposis colon cancer (HNPCC) (Autosomal dominant)

3. **Immuno deficiency Syndrome**

    e.g.
    - Agammaglobulinemia – X – linked
    - Wiskott-Aldrich Syndrome-autosomal recessive

4. **Monogenic predisposition to neoplasia**
    - Tylosis (Keratosis palmaris et plantaris) with esophageal cancer
    - α - antitrypsium deficiency – hepatocellular carcinoma

Several Mendelian syndromes are known associated with a high-risk of malignancy, and many of these genes have been mapped and even cloned (see Table 12.C).

The retinoblastoma gene specifies a 10-kilodalton protein (p105) found in the nucleus and is a suppressor of DNA transcription. It binds with at least three known oncogene proteins: the EIA protein of adenovirus, the SV40 large T antigen, and the 16E7 protein of human papilloma virus, a virus associated with 50% of cervical carcinomas. This implies that these three viruses use a similar mechanism in transformation, and this mechanism may involve inactivation of the retinoblastoma p105 protein.

A third tumour-suppressor gene is the p53 gene which has been implicated in a wide range of cancers including leukaemia, carcinomas of the lung and breast, brain tumours, bone cancers and soft-tissue sarcomas found in human cancers. The gene is located in band p13 of chromosome 17.

Table 12.C. Cloned Genes In Dominantly Inherited Cancers

DISORDER	Gene symbol	Gene type	Chromosomal localisation
Basal cell nevus syndrome	BCNS	TS	9q31
Familial adenomatous polyposis	APC	TS	5q21
Familial breast-ovarian cancer	BRCA1	TS	17q21
	BRCA2	TS	13q12-13
Familial melanoma	MLM	TS	9q21
Li-Fraumeni syndrome	P53	TS	17p13
Multiple endocrine neoplasia 2A	MEN2A	Onc	10q11
Neurofibromatosis type 1	NF1	TS	17q11
Neurofibromatosis type 2	NF2	TS	22q12
Retinoblastoma	RBI	TS	13q14
Tuberous sclerosis	TSC2	TS	16p13
Von Hippel-Lindau disease	VHL	TS	3p25
Wilms's tumour	WT1	TS	11p13

* TS= tumour suppressor, Onc=oncogene.
From Knudson AG. All in the (cancer) family. Nature Genetics 1993; 5: 103-4.

Chromosome Rearrangements and Cancer

For many years, it has been known that certain types of cancers are associated with chromosomal rearrangements. For example, chronic myelogenous leukaemia (CML) in human beings is associated with an aberration involving chromosomes 9 and 22. This abnormal chromosome was originally discovered in the city of Philadelphia, and thus is called the **Philadelphia chromosome**. Initially, it was thought to have a simple deletion in its long arm; however, subsequent analysis using molecular techniques has shown that the Philadelphia chromosome is actually involved in a reciprocal translocation with chromosome 9. In this translocation, the tip of the long arm of chromosome 9 gets joined to the body of chromosome 22, and the distal portion of the long arm of chromosome 22 gets exchanged to the body of chromosome 9. The translocation breakpoint on chromosome 9 is in the *c-abl* oncogene, and the breakpoint on chromosome 22 is in a gene called *bcr*, which encodes a tyrosine kinase. Through the translocation, the *bcr* and *c-abl* genes have been physically joined, creating a fusion gene whose polypeptide product has the amino terminus of the *bcr* protein and the carboxy terminus of the *abl* protein. The fusion protein is a strong marker of carcinogenesis in CML, apart from some other leukemias.

Burkitt's lymphoma is another example of a white cell cancer associated with reciprocal translocations. These translocations invariably involve chromosome 8 and one of the three chromosomes (2, 14, and 22) that carry genes encoding immunoglobulins. Translocations involving chromsomes

8 and 14 are the most common. In these translocations, the *c-myc* oncogene on chromosome 8 is juxtaposed to the genes for the immunoglobulin heavy chains on chromosome 14. As a result of this rearrangement, the *c-myc* gene is overexpressed in cells that produce immunoglobulin heavy chains, that is, in B lymphocytes, and this overexpression causes the cells to become cancerous (Table 12.D).

Table 12.D. Examples of Proto-Oncogenes Implicated In Human Malignancy

Proto-oncogene	Molecular abnormality	Disorder
myc	Translocation 8q24	Burkitt's lymphoma
abl	Translocation 9q34	Chronic myeloid leukaemia
mos	Translocation 8q22	Acute myeloid leukaemia
myc	Amplification	Carcinoma of breast, lung, cervix, oesophagus
		Neuroblastoma, small cell carcinoma of lung
N-myc	Amplification	Carcinoma of colon, lung, and pancreas;
K-ras	Point mutation	melanoma
		Carcinomas of genitourinary tract, thyroid
H-ras	Point mutation	

Familial cancer syndromes are of two types -

1) Li-Fraumeni syndrome due to somatic mutations in p53 tumour suppressor gene affects colon, stomach, pancreas, breast, endometrium, and genitourinary tract.

Lung cancers often show somatic mutations of the retinoblastoma (RB) gene, but this tumour does not occur in individuals who inherit germline RB mutations. These genes may play a greater part in progression of tumours than in initiation of the cancer.

2) Lynch type 2, due to mutations in 4 genes involved in mismatch DNA repairs affects colon, breast, sarcoma brain, leukaemia, adrenal cells etc. Autosomal dominant genes with 80-90% penetrance so that 40% probands develop associated cancers. Mutations in repair genes predispose the individual to cancer, not all people necessarily develop tumors.

In Lynch cancer family syndrome type 2 (LCFS2) a proportion of cases are linked to a gene on chromosome 2. However, the colonic cancers commonly associated with LCFS2 show somatic mutations similar to those found in sporadic colon cancers, that is in the adenomatous polyposis coli (APC), oncogene K-ras, tumour suppressor p53, and deleted–in-colon-cancer (DCC) genes. LCFS2 gene on chromosome 2 may be acting as a tumour suppressor gene.

Tumour-Suppressor Genes

Tumor-suppressor genes (anti-cancer or **anti-oncogenes**) act by suppressing malignant growth; in the homozygous recessive state, however, cancer ensues. The first tumor-suppressor gene to be isolated was the gene for **retinoblastoma**, a tumor of retinoblast cells, which are precursors to cone cells in the retina of the eye. This is a disease of young children because after the retinoblast cells differentiate, they no longer divide and apparently can no longer form tumors. The disease occurs both in hereditary and a sporadic form. Both forms are presumably due to the recessive homozygous or, hemizygous states. In the hereditary form, individuals inherit one mutant allele; a second mutation generates the disease. In the sporadic form (with identical symptoms), apparently both alleles mutate spontaneously in the somatic tissue of the retina. Alfred Knudson (1971) suggested that two mutations are required for retinoblastoma. In addition, the retinoblastoma gene has also been implicated in other cancers including sarcomas and carcinomas of the lung, bladder, and breast.

Yunis examined the cells from several retinoblastoma patients and found that there was frequent deletion of chromosome 13, specifically band q14, on the longer arm of the chromosome. He noticed that the exact points of deletion varied from patient to patient indicating the loss of gene action rather than enhancement of gene activity as responsible for the outcome.

Further support of tumor-suppressor genes was provided from studies on another childhood cancer, **Wilm's tumor,** a kidney cancer that is also believed to be caused by the loss of activity of a tumor-suppressor gene which is associated with the loss of band p13 on short arm of chromosome 11. Researchers introduced a normal chromosome 11 into Wilm's tumor cells growing in culture and this resulted in normal cell growth, exactly what would be predicted if the normal gene was a tumor-suppressor.

Tumorigenesis is a multistage process and involves both oncogenes and tumour suppressor genes. The common altered gene in human cancers is the tumour suppressor gene p53, which occurs in about 70% of all tumours, whereas mutations in the RAS oncogene occur in about one-third of all cancers. Inherited forms of the common cancers, for example breast cancer, constitutes about 5% of all breast cancer cases, and is one of the most common of all genetic cancers. The hereditary breast cancer locus (BRCA1) on chromosome 17q is implicated in all hereditary breast and ovarian cancers. In several cancers like the colorectal carcinomas, DNA repair errors are particularly known to play an etiological role. Mismatch repair gene errors were found to be attributable often to microsatellite instability in the genome in almost all tissue cancer types (Vasavi et al, 2016). Repair gene methylation errors are reported in hMLH1, hMSH2, PMS1 etc. while mutations in repair genes like BRCA1 and BRCA2 are reported.

Targeted cancer therapies act upon specific genes and proteins that promote cancer in a particular tissue. Different studies have been conducted and several types of targeted therapy are in practice. Monoclonal antibodies, for instance may block a specific target outside the cancer cell or may be used to direct toxic substances (chemotherapeutic agent) to it. Small molecule drugs like angiogenesis inhibitors block the processes that prevent the spread of cancer, by starving the tumor of new blood vessels. Then there are tumor agonistic treatments that are not specific to a type of cancer but act upon specific genetic changes that contribute to the cancer process. These therapies are often used in combination with traditional chemotherapy and radiation to get the desired effect and tumor reduction, resulting in the patient showing good prognosis.

CHAPTER 13 Radiation Genetics

Radiation may come from either an external source, such as an x-ray machine, or an internal source, such as an injected radioisotope. An overview may help explain not only the effects of radiation but also the motivation for studying them, which led too much of the research. Mavor, hundred years ago showed that X-rays could produce genetic changes both by increasing number of crossing over, an increased incidence of chromosomal non-disjunction during cell division. H.J. Muller, in 1927, studied estimating mutations and number of secondary linked mutations. This discovery fetched him the Nobel Prize. Radiation is the emission or transmission of energy in the form of waves or particles through space or through a material medium. It includes:

1. Ionizing radiation: Higher Ultraviolet radiation, X-ray, Gamma radiation, Alpha radiation, Beta radiation, Neutron radiation.
2. Cosmic radiation: Cosmic radiation consists of high-energy charged particles, x-rays and gamma rays produced in space.
3. Non-Ionizing radiation: Lower Ultraviolet light, Visible, light, Infrared, Microwave, Radio waves, Very low frequency radiations , Extremely low frequency, Thermal radiation (heat), Black-body radiation.

Ionizing radiation, "ionizes" that means, pushes an electron out of its orbit around an atomic nucleus, causing the formation of electrical charges on atoms or molecules. If this electron comes from the DNA itself or from a neighboring molecule and directly strikes and disrupts the DNA molecule, the effect is called direct action. This initial ionization takes place very quickly, in about 0.000000000000001 (1×10^{-15}) of a second. However, today it is estimated that about two-thirds of the damage caused by X-rays is due to indirect action.

Non-ionizing radiations - Exposure to electromagnetic fields in this frequency range can warm up exposed tissues because these absorb the radio wave and microwave energy and convert these into heat. The frequency level determines the depth of penetration into the body. Warming up by this radiation is the most dangerous for the brain, eyes, genitals, stomach, liver and kidneys. How deep the radiation penetrates depends on the frequency. If resonances occur in parts of the body then the damage can increase. Worldwide the maximum acceptable radiation level varies from 10 mW/cm² to 0.1 mW/cm².

Cosmic radiation' usually refers specifically to the cosmic microwave background radiation. This consists of very, very low energy photons (energy of about 2.78 Kelvin) whose spectrum is peaked in the microwave region and which are remnants from the time when the universe was only about 200,000 years old. These higher energy particles are potentially dangerous, but most of these particles never make it to the earth. They are deflected by magnetic fields between us and the source, or they interact with other particles, or they decay in flight. Here is only one type of cosmic radiation known to adversely affect us and that's UV radiation from our sun, which causes skin cancer in millions of people every year. Again, our atmosphere serves as a shield, but ultraviolet photons do make it through and without that protective ozone layer which blocks these photons, we are going to need cosmetic protective lotions that currently are in use.

Possible damage to Health and Environment from certain types of radiation:

The impact of radiation on living tissue is complicated by the type of radiation and the variety of tissues. In addition, the effects of radiation are not always easy to separate from other factors, making it a challenge at times for scientists to isolate them. Although powerful methods such as whole-genome-sequencing techniques have become available to detect radiation effects in human germ cells, the mutation induction rate in the genome now appears to be much lower than was previously thought. Consequently, detecting radiation effects in human germ cells still remains a difficult task.

1. Radiation induced mutagenesis
2. Ultraviolet radiations and mutations
3. Effect of radiations on populations

How can ionizing radiation produce genetic mutations?

Radiation may alter the DNA within any cell. Cell damage and death that result from mutations in somatic cells occur only in the organism in which the mutation occurred and are therefore termed somatic or non-heritable effects. Cancer is the most notable long-term somatic effect. In contrast, mutations that occur in germ cells (sperm and ova) can be transmitted to future generations and are therefore called genetic or heritable effects. Genetic effects may not appear until many generations later. The genetic effects of radiation were first demonstrated in fruit flies in the 1920s. Genetic mutation due to radiation simply produces a greater frequency of the same mutations that occur continuously and spontaneously in nature. Like cancers, the genetic effects of radiation are impossible to distinguish from mutations due to other causes. Today at least 1,300 diseases are known to be caused by a mutation. Some mutations may be beneficial; random mutation is the driving force in evolution. In contrast to estimates of cancer risk, which are based in part on studies of human populations, estimates of heritable risk are based for the most part upon animal studies.

Given the lack of direct evidence of any increase in human heritable (genetic) effects resulting from radiation exposure, the estimates of genetic risks in humans have been compared with experimental data obtained with laboratory animals. However, estimates of human genetic risks vary greatly from animal data. For example, fruit flies have very large chromosomes that appear to be uniquely susceptible to radiation. Humans may be less vulnerable than previously thought. Statistical lower limits on the doubling dose have been calculated that are compatible with the observed human data. Based on our inability to demonstrate an effect in humans, the lower limit for the genetic doubling dose is thought to be less than 100 rem.

The risk of genetic mutation is expressed in terms of the doubling dose: the amount of radiation that would cause additional mutations equal in number to those that already occurring naturally from all causes, thereby doubling the naturally occurring rate of mutation. It is generally believed that mutation rates depend linearly on dose and that there is no threshold below which mutation rates would not be increased. Spontaneous mutation (unrelated to radiation) occurs naturally at a rate of approximately 1/10,000 to 1/1,000,000 cell divisions per gene, with wide variation from one gene to another. Attempts have been made to estimate the contribution of ionizing radiation to human mutation rates by studying offspring of both exposed and unexposed Japanese atomic bomb survivors. These estimates are based on comparisons of the rate of various congenital defects and cancer between exposed and unexposed survivors, as well as on direct counting of mutations at a small number of genes. For all these endpoints, no excess has been observed among descendants of the exposed survivors.

How can radiation cause cancer?

Cancer is produced if radiation does not kill the cell but creates an error in the DNA blueprint that contributes to eventual loss of control of cell division, and the cell begins dividing uncontrollably. This effect might not appear for many years. Cancers induced by radiation do not differ from cancers due to other causes, so there is no simple way to measure the rate of cancer due to radiation. Studies of irradiated animals and exposed groups of people have yielded better estimates of the risk of cancer due to radiation. This type of research is complicated by the variety of cancers, which vary in radio sensitivity. For example, bone marrow is more sensitive than skin cells to radiation-induced cancer. Large doses of radiation to large numbers of people are needed in order to cause measurable increases in the number of cancers and thus determine the differences in the sensitivity of different organs to radiation. Because the cancers can occur anytime in the exposed person's lifetime, these studies can take seventy years or more to complete. For example, the largest and scientifically most valuable epidemiologic study of radiation effects has been the ongoing study of the Japanese Atomic bomb survivors. Other important studies include studies of large groups exposed to radiation as a consequence of their occupation (such as uranium miners) or as a consequence of medical treatment.

Human exposure to radiation comes from less known sources like building material such as sandstone, brick, gypsum, granite or from medical tests we undergo maybe even an airport security scanner. The only way to combat these exposures would be to limit heavy doses where possible and maintain a healthy lifestyle and diet to correct genetic errors that may be harmful.

CHAPTER 14
Orofacial Genetic Disorders

Orofacial clefts are common congenital malformations of the lip, palate, or both caused by complex genetic and environmental factors. Each of these conditions emerges by the disruption of distinct morphogenetic processes at different stages of embryological development. Males are more likely than females to have a cleft lip with or without cleft palate, while females are at a slightly greater risk for cleft palate alone. Developmental tooth abnormalities, including mild and more severe forms of tooth agenesis, have often been reported in patients affected with orofacial clefts. Since facial mesenchyme is derived from neural crest, it is postulated that periconceptional folic acid supplementation may reduce the occurrence of offspring with orofacial clefts. Zinc also is important in fetal development, and deficiency of this nutrient causes isolated cleft palate and other malformations. Therefore manipulation of maternal lifestyle with improved use of multivitamins and other supplements can be preventive strategies. The inheritance of these conditions may be single-gene inheritance as a result of a single gene carried by one parent and the multifactorial inheritance as a result of a number of genetic and nongenetic factors, such as alcohol, drugs, and environmental factors that can be causative.

While prenatal diagnosis of cleft is readily attainable using conventional 2D sonography, however, cleft palate is more difficult to identify especially if it is an associated anomaly. Minor clefts (e.g., submucus cleft palate and bifid uvula) might not be diagnosed until later in life. Inclusion of 3D and 4D ultrasound imaging allows easier and more precise evaluation of the different cleft constituents. Prenatal diagnosis involves a series of methods and procedures that can diagnose defect, malformation or hereditary disease during pregnancy. This gives parents the advantage of having time to prepare emotionally for the birth and become knowledgeable about the birth defect. Cleft lip or palate can be seen as an associated feature in ≥300 syndromes where specific genes are implicated in the etiology. Gene identification for non-syndromic cleft lip and palate is difficult because of the varying levels of its penetrance, sex differences, and other environmental factors.

The Meckel–Gruber syndrome is the most severe form of the autosomal recessive ciliopathies and is characterized by the presence of posterior cephaloceles, polycystic kidneys, and polydactyly; it is also frequently accompanied by facial clefts and microphthalmia/anophthalmia. Less severe ciliopathies including Joubert's syndrome and oral–facial–digital syndrome type IV may also be associated to a lesser extent with facial dysmorphism, cleft lip and palate, and facial tumors. Anterior cephalocele has been described in fetuses with frontonasal dysplasia (FND), also known as median cleft facial syndrome. This condition is usually sporadic, but autosomal dominant, recessive, and X-linked patterns, as well as 22q11 microdeletion are reported. Severe forms of FND, particularly when involving the brain, may be associated with autosomal recessive mutations in aristaless-like homeobox gene ALX1 where ALX1 expression is essential for building oral and nasal cavities as well as proper eye development during early embryogenesis. The association between open neural tube defects and facial anomalies appears to be sporadic and not related to any known syndrome.

The Hapsburg Jaw

The Hapsburg jaw is a Royal dominant trait with incomplete penetrance and variable expression. During the Middle Ages to the last century, the house of Hapsburg ruled much of the Europe. The members included kings, queens, emperors, and empresses. Although the Hapsburg power was concentrated in Central Europe, especially Austriat, various times in history it encompasses Spain, the Low Countries and some parts of Italy. The extension of Hapsburg power was due in part, to the family's uncanny ability to arrange politically beneficial marriages. This skill is well celebrated in the following translation of Latin into English, *"Let others wage wars, you happy Austria, marry"*. Thus, through a foreign policy that was based on matrimonial vows, the Hapsburg spread genes among European nobility, Marie Antoinette, wife of French king Louis XVI for example, was a Hapsburg.

As the Hapsburg spread their genes, so did, they spread the phenotypes associated with those genes. The most famous of these phenotypes is the Hapsburg jaws, a curious potting idiosyncrasy protrusion of the lower lip and unusually the lower jaw protrude, sometimes forcing the mouth partly open, the mandible associated with difficulty in chewing. This condition is better known as mandibular prognathism. Its presence is well recorded in paintings, sculptures, coins and of late in photographs. Considered as an excellent example of the long persistence of dominant genes, this oddity has also appeared in the faces of some Hapsburg women; one of them was Maria Terresa, Queen of Hungary and Bohemia in the 18th century.

Orofacial Genetic Disorders | 121

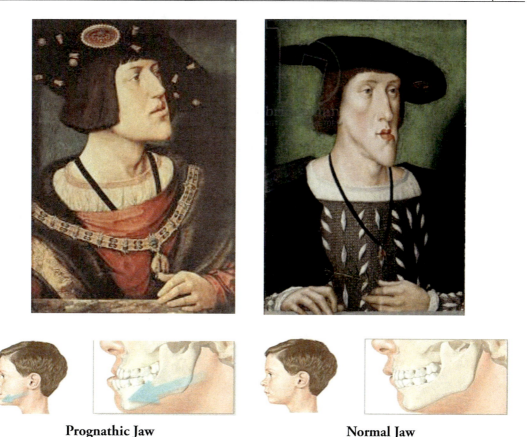

Prognathic Jaw   **Normal Jaw**

Figure 14.1: Images showing Hapsburg women with the prognatic jaw, skeletal image depicting a comparison with a normal jaw.

The best documented case of prognathism among the Hapsburg appears in portraits of the emperor Kaiser Maximillan I of Austria (1459-1519). Maximillan's son, Philip I, married Joanna, the daughter of King Ferdinand and Queen Isabela of Spain. In this way, Phillip I became king of Spain and established a Spanish line of Hapsburg. It is not known whether Philip I manifested the Hapsburg jaw, his son Charles V (1500-1558) clearly had prognathism that caused his mouth to hang open and had difficulty in chewing food. His son Philip IV clearly had prognatic jaw and because of shyness in political realm, he handed over the government of Spain to professional politicians. The Spanish line of Hapsburgs ended with his son's Carlos ll death in 1700.

Five hundred years of Hapsburg portraiture clearly indicates that mandibular prognathism is caused by a dominant allele with incomplete penetrance and variable expression of this condition has been found to varying degrees in couple of dozen members of the Hapsburg families,

The portraits of both men and women clearly show (see Figure 14.1) the condition although the mode of inheritance is typical for that of dominant allele. Rarely this condition skips a generation presumably because the dominant allele is not fully penetrant. The physiological and other related aspects are currently unknown although worth pursuing as their ancestors must be there either in Austria and Hungary.

15

CHAPTER

Sex Determination in Humans

In many species, definitely including the humans, sex differentiation is genetic where the male and female have a specific set of chromosomes that describe their sexual development. Meiosis is the process in which sex cells divide and create new sex cells with half the number of chromosomes. Sperms and eggs are sex cells with each cell contributing 23 pairs of chromosomes. If meiosis does not take place normally and there are errors in segregation, the fetus may have extra or less than normal number of chromosomes.

Advanced maternal age is an important risk factor where the couple is at a risk of having a baby with a chromosomal abnormality (Figure 15-1a). This is because the errors in meiosis may be more likely to happen with increasing age in them (Figure 15-1b). Women's eggs begin to mature at puberty while men make new sperms as an ongoing process so age-based risk doesn't affect as much (Figure 15-1c & d). Though there are abnormalities for the fetus from older fathers too. Certain types of morphologically abnormal spermatozoa, such as macrocephalic multitailed spermatozoa, are associated with a very significantly increased frequency of aneuploidy. Basic chromosomal proteins in mammalian sperm (protamines) were drastically different from proteins of somatic cells (histones). During pregnancy, exposure of the mother to medicines, alcohol, radiation or certain health conditions may raise the risk for a birth defect in a baby.

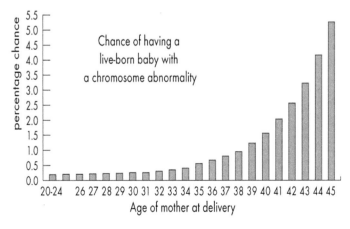

(a)

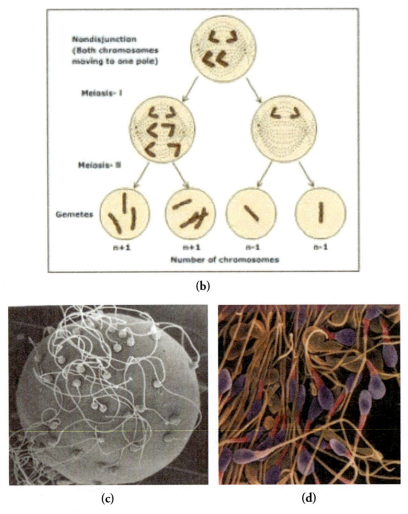

Figure 15-1 (a) Increased risk of having a child with a chromosomal abnormality with increased mother's age (b) Chromosomal meiotic segregation errors leading to progeny with abnormal chromosome number (c) Mature eggs with sperms in process of fertilization where the egg bears the age of the female (d) New sperm production is an ongoing process in the males

The Y chromosome

The Y chromosome named by Wilson, 1909 is found in eukaryotic organism with male heterogeneity and diploid sex including insects, mammals, plants etc. and in combination with X chromosome, forms the most common XY sex determining system. The X & Y chromosomes are not strictly homologous; the homology is about 5% only. The Y chromosome is much smaller than X and carries lesser genes, nevertheless, during meiosis, behave as homologues so that gametes produced by males are either the X or Y chromosome.

The Y chromosome is one of sex chromosomes and is grouped under the category of **G** acrocentric chromosomes and devoid of satellite and has a very short **p** arm and slightly bigger **q** arm. With fluorescent banding technique, the longer arm fluoresces and with quinacrine hydrochloride, the Y chromosome brightly fluoresces. Its transmission is holandric i.e., inheritance is from fathers to sons. The presence of Y measures about 2 µ in length and slightly longer than rest of the chromosomes of G group i.e.21, 22. The Y chromosome ensures maleness irrespective of the number of X chromosomes as in XXY, XXXY etc. It is the smallest chromosome and devoid of satellites in the human genome and known to contain 86 to 231 genes coding 23 distinct proteins only and almost all are male determining, male fertility and represents 2-3% of haploid human genome.

Y chromosome has a complex structure and about 5% of the chromosome recombines with homologous sequences on the X chromosome (Figure 15-2). This is called the **p**seudo **a**utosomal **r**egion (PAR), which is present at both the ends, the distal end is PAR 1 and the proximal is PAR 2. This region has several genes, the most important are *MIC2*, *SRY* (sex determining region) and *ZFY* (Zinc Finger protein) and *AZF1* (azoospermic factor). The remainder of the chromosome is inactive heterochromatic and does not recombine with any other chromosome and is called as **n**on**-r**ecombining region on **Y** (NRY). The NRY is 60mb in size, of which only 35 mb is euchromatic that consists of highly repetitive unique DNA rich in transposons. The repeats may be short or long. Two major tandem repeat sequences, *DYZ1* and *DYZ2* are organised in large arrays in the heterochromatic region of the long arm. The *DYZ1* has 3000 copies while *DYZ2* has 2000 copies. However, there are small numbers of expressed genes that fall into three classes.

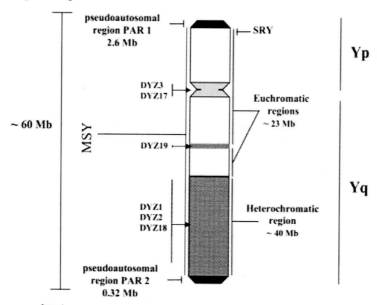

Figure 15-2: Structure of Y-chromosome

There are eight class I genes that have homologues on the X chromosome and are widely expressed throughout the body. There are also eight class ll genes which are expressed only in the testis and do not have homologues on the X chromosome. The five class lll genes have homologues on the X chromosome but show tissue limited expression, which in three cases is confined to the testes. The *SRY* region that determines male sexual development is located on the class ll genes and is expressed only in the embryonic bipotential gonad and in the adult testes. Its homologue on the X chromosome is called *SOX3,* which is active and presumably performs some other essential functions in both male and female functions. As most of the Y chromosome consists of number of non-recombining region, the mapping of genes is done by deletion mapping. The entire length of the Y chromosome has been divided into seven deletion intervals; intervals 1, 2, 3 are on short **p** arm while intervals 5, 6, 7 are on long **q** arm extending up to the centromere. Each of these deletion intervals have been further divided into sub-intervals A, B, C etc.

The Y chromosome shows very little sequence variation which in part may be due to its low effective population size which is just one quarter that of the autosomal region. The Y chromosome also shows polymorphism and this will not be discussed here.

The term Y linked is used to refer to loci found only on Y chromosome which controls holandric traits/inheritance. Y chromosome SRY is responsible for testes development /formation, production of testosterone and for secondary sexual characteristics. It was showed that Y linked inheritance is the presence of hairs on the pinna of the ear called as Hypertrichosis pinnae auris. In addition, there are also some non-functional genes on the Y chromosome, such as the genes for height (XYY men are taller than XY), gene for steroidal sulphatase, a gene for tooth growth, a gene for the Kallmann syndrome, a disease of gonadal and olfactory functions. Further, a gene for speed maturation and the non-functional genes similar to the genes for the protein actin and the enzyme arginosuccinate also found. Y linked diseases are rare, however, Y chromosome deletions of SRY gene frequently causes male sterility due to defective testicular development. Y chromosome polysomy (i.e. XYY, XYYY, XYYYY) especially the latter is rare and such patients have low IQ with skeletal abnormalities. In the past it was thought that persons with extra Y chromosome are antisocial, with abnormal criminal behavior and dubbed as "Criminal karyotype". However, this concept is incorrect and obsolete.

About 300 milllion years ago, the Y chromosome was made up of 1400 genes as against 45 genes reported to be preset now. If this depletion of genes continues the Y chromosome will be defunct in the next 4-5 million years or even less. The Y chromosome determines maleness and male fertility. If this happens how the human species without men survive!

The X-Chromosome

This was first observed and named so by Wilson 1906. Historically it was T.H. Morgan who first noted in 1910 white eyed *Drosophila* mutants which on crossing with wild (red) gave red eyed F_1 progeny which on back crossing gave 1/2 each red and ½ white eyed Drosophila. This was an important finding and lends support to the chromosome theory of inheritance. Thus, X is denoted for wild type and X⁺ for the mutant. X chromosomes are group of chromosomes (multiple X) in eukaryotes especially mammals and humans, and with a feature of basic heterogametic/heteromorphic sex determination system since the X and Y chromosomes are dissimilar. Sex linked genes means genes/loci present on the X chromosomes in contrast to those present on Y chromosomes and are called Y linked.

The X chromosome is one of the sex determining and part of the XY sex determination system. The chromosome was named for its unique properties by earlier workers and its counterpart is Y chromosome. The X chromosome a large sub-metacentric chromosome with medium length about 5.0 to 5.5 um depending on the preparation and intermediate between chromosomes 7 and 8 and belongs the C group of chromosomes. It has large number of genes on both the arms. With the development of fluorescent banding techniques, visual differentiation of the X chromosomes and morphologically similar to some autosomes became clear.

Normally, the female has two XX while the male has only one X chromosome, and this creates imbalance of the ratio of X linked genes in two sexes. To compensate for this difference, one randomly selected X chromosome is inactivated (X inactivation also called Lyonisation). X inactivation is passed on to all future somatic cells and there is evidence that X inactivation also occurs randomly in embryonic cells. This was worked out by Mary Lyon and Liane Russell in 1961 independently. Lyon proposed that dosage compensation in mammals including humans occurs by the inactivation of X chromosome in females. These observations brought to light the evidence from cytological study by Murray Barr and Evert Bertram (1949) form Canada that a highly condensed structure in the interphase nuclei of somatic cells of female cats that was absent in male cats.

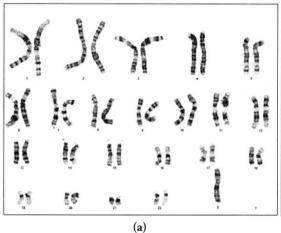

(a)

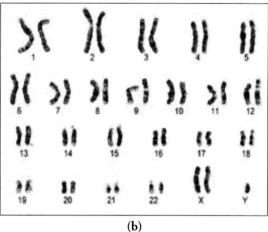

(b)

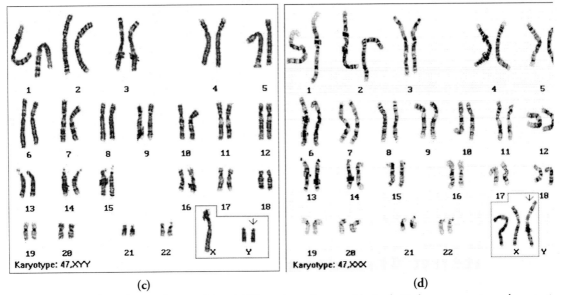

Figure 15-3 Sex chromosome abnormalities: (a) Turner's syndrome with single X chromosome in a phenotypic female (b) Klinefelter's syndrome with XXY karyotype (c) Additional Y chromosome making the chromosome number 47, XYY (d) 47, XXX karyotype in female

This heterochromatic body is transcriptionally inactive X chromosome (most of the genes are inactive and not expressed) and this body can be seen by light microscope as a distinct structure called the Barr body which is located near the nuclear membrane and replicates late in S phase, was confirmed by Ohno in 1960. The number of Barr bodies in females is directly related to the number of X chromosomes. Barr body is absent in males and Turner's syndrome females (XY, XO), one Barr body is present in normal female and abnormal male (XX, XXY), two Barr bodies are present in abnormal female and abnormal male (XXX, XXXY) and three Barr bodies present in abnormal female (XXXX). Bar bodies equals the number of inactivated X chromosome. Figure 15-3 shows various sex chromosome anomalies that differ from the normal male (XY) or female (XX) chromosome set.

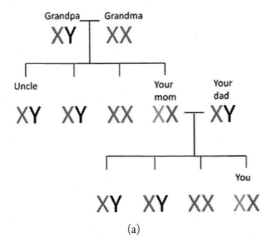

(a)

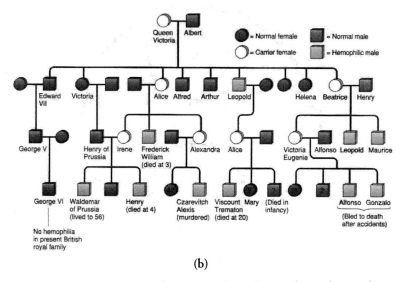

Figure 15.4 (a) Pedigree showing inheritance of colour blindness (b) A pedigree showing hemophilia in Queen Victoria family

Once the gene is found to be X linked, determination of the position of the locus on the X chromosome and to determine map unit between loci is important. As shown in figure 15.4a, if the trait for colour blindness is found in father, the grandson will have the trait, hence called as "**grandfather method**". Some of the common X linked traits are Duchenne Muscular dystrophy (DMD), Fragile-X syndrome, Haemophilia A & B and testicular feminization although the list is long. The famous case of inheritance of Hemophilia in the Royal family of Queen Victoria is shown in pedigree Figure 15.4b. In addition red-green colour blindness and anhidrotic ectodermal dysplasia also show X linked inheritance.

16 Dermatoglyphics
CHAPTER

The term Dermatoglyphics (derma= skin, glyph=carving) was introduced by Cummins (1926) to describe ridge patterns on palm skin, digits and foot soles and he collected fingerprint patterns amongst various racial groups and established the relative frequency. Later Cummins and Midlo referred this condition as "***poor man's karyotype***". However, it was Sir Francis Galton, the cousin of Charles Darwin who first classified fingerprints patterns as, ***arches*** with no triradius as significant indicator of fingerprint pattern type in addition to ***loops*** with one triradius, radial, and ulner loops that opens on the radial or ulnar side of the finger and ***whorled*** with two triradii patterns. His two works on Fingerprints dated 1892 and 1895 are considered as classics in the field of early dermatoglypics and are vastly used by anthropologists, geneticists, and criminologists. Study of dermatoglyphics is important in medical genetics mainly because of the characteristic combinations of pattern types associated with some chromosomal disorders and syndromes since these patterns are heritable. Specific patterns have been seen to be prevalent in specific tribes and sub-populations (Prasannalatha et al, 1997). Furthermore, the study of dermatoglyphics is routinely used as one of the methods of measuring resemblances between twins in the determination of twin zygosity. The ridge count expresses the size of the finger pattern and the number of ridges between triradius to the core of the pattern. When the triradius is absent, the arch count is zero while the sum of the ridge counts of 10 fingers is called total ridge count. The trait is polygenic and inherited.

Cummins and Midlo's work inspired L.S. Penrosehair of Eugenics, London University dermatoglyphic research on hands of the patients with Down's syndrome such as mongolism related trisomies, Edward's syndrome and Patau's syndrome and also initiated rare chromosomal disorders such as Cri du Chat syndrome and the sex chromosome disorders such as Turner's and Kleinefelter's syndrome (Figure 16.1). Based on the information, he concluded that the hand revealed particular malformations peculiar to these conditions and hence diagnostic.

In 1965, the Galton Laboratory was renamed as "Kenedt-Galton Centre for Clinical Genetics and Mental deficiency" dedicated to chromosomal and dermatoglyphic research and also offering genetic counseling for prospective parents. Penrose pioneered in developing number of dermatoglyphic methodical procedures and practices. It was he that formulated the measurement to establish the position of the displaced axial triradius in terms of ATD angles shown in Figure 16.1 as well as for establishing the inheritance of its position in the palm. Siamian crease is fairly a common feature found in 50% of Down's cases, and single crease on the fifth finger axial triradius in the centre of the palm with wide gap between the first and second toe.

Plantar (feet)) patterns, sole, tibial arch pattern in hallucal area are associated with Down's syndrome patients. Dermatoglyphic data support investigation for completing a diagnosis and is also useful in criminology. No wonder fingerprints of thumbs and off late the entire palm and sole are used as useful markers for identifying persons in census data. Sarah Holt, Penrose's assistant's work "the *Genetics of Dermal Ridges*" published in 1968 provides comprehensive review. Schaumann and Alters (1976) book on "*Dermatoglyphics in medical disorders*" provides useful additional information to those interested in the subject.

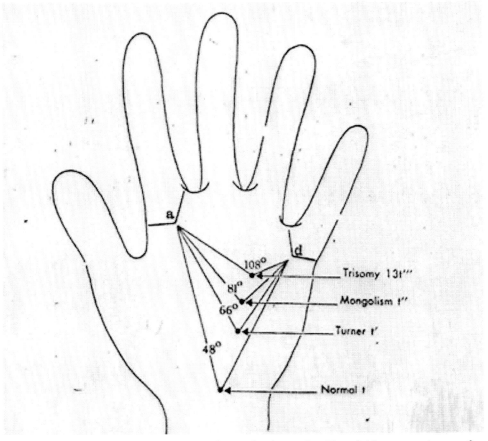

Figure 16-1: Dermatoglyphics - Mean position of most distal tri-radius T in children up to 4 years of age.

Medical dermatoglyphics deals with diagnosis of various illnesses including schizophrenia and leukemia and the experts claim a very high degree of accuracy in their prognostics ability from the hands features alone. In Germany the subject of dermatoglyphics has been taken up seriously to the extent of computer programs have been designed to perform rapid multivariate assessments of new born developing heart disease, cancer, diabetes, and mental illness. It's heartening that dermatoglyphics is an integral part of medical syllabus in many German universities.

17 Linkage and Gene Mapping

CHAPTER

Linkage is a condition in which two or more non allelic genes tend to be inherited together. Linked genes have their loci along the same chromosome and do not assort independently but can be separated by crossing over. Linked genes tend to remain together in passing from one generation to the next. The strength of linkage between 2 pairs of genes varies inversely with the amount of recombination or crossing over between them. The strength of the linkage is same whether linkage is measured in cis/trans phase (coupling/repulsion phase). Sex linkage is the pattern of inheritance resulting from genes located on the sex chromosomes.

The group of genes that have their loci on the same chromosome is called linkage group. Measurement of genetic linkage is expressed as centimorgan unit (cM) or percent recombination i.e. if loci are separated by crossing over in 1% of gametes which are 1 cM apart.

Mapping human genes is critically important for a number of reasons. Knowledge of genes and their location gives us insight into the evolutionary relationship of humans to other primates. Equally important is, mapping the disease genes creates an opportunity for researchers to isolate the gene and understand how it causes a disease. In subsequent cases, researchers have mapped a gene to a specific chromosome, and then proceeded to isolate the gene for further study. Duchenne muscular dystrophy, cystic fibrosis, Huntington's disease, and breast cancer are examples of the success of mapping disease genes to specific regions of specific chromosomes and subsequently isolating those genes.

Until recently, mapping genes in humans has been difficult. It was complicated by the fact that it is not possible to make the controlled crosses which is common with *Drosphila*. However, in spite of the limitations, there are several ways to analyse linkage in humans.

The oldest and most direct way to ascertain linkage relationships in humans is the analysis of pedigrees. By itself, this is a cumbersome strategy. However, when pedigree analysis is coupled with modern molecular and somatic cell genetic techniques, researchers acquire important insights into the arrangement of genes on human chromosomes

Human Pedigrees

The analysis of segregation by this method is not possible in human beings because matings cannot be controlled on ethical reasons. However, the mode of inheritance of a trait can sometimes be determined by examining the segregation of alleles in several generations of related individuals. This is typically done with a family tree that shows the phenotype of each individual member; such a diagram is called a pedigree. An important application of *Probability* in genetics is its use in pedigree analysis. By analysing the pedigree, we may be able to determine how the gene controlling the trait is inherited.

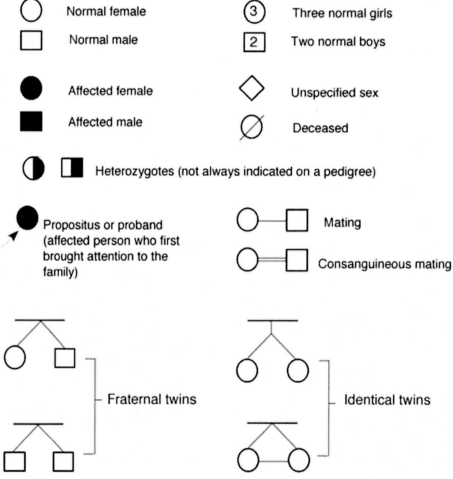

Figure: 17.1 Symbols used in pedigree analysis

As stated in Figure 17.1, the conventions used in constructing a pedigree are shown. Circles represent females, and squares designate males. If the sex is unknown, a diamond may be used. If a pedigree traces only a single trait, the circles, squares, and diamonds are shaded, if the phenotype being considered is expressed. Heterozygotes who fail to express a recessive trait, when known with certainty, have only the right half of their square or circle shaded.

The parents are connected by a horizontal line, and vertical lines lead to their offspring. All such offspring are called sibs and are connected by a horizontal sibship line. Sibs are placed from left to right according to birth order and are labeled with Arabic numerals. Each generation is indicated by a Roman numeral.

Twins are indicated by connected diagonal lines. Monozygotic or identical twins stem from a single line itself connected to the sibship line. Dizygotic or fraternal twins are connected directly to the sibship line. A number within one of the symbols represents numerous sibs of the same or unknown phenotypes. A male whose phenotype drew the attention of a physician or geneticist is called the propositus (a female is a proposita) or sometimes the proband and is indicated by an arrow Unlike other organisms, linkage in humans is studied differently.

- Linkage in family is calculated by Lod Score, proposed by Newton E. Morton which is acronym for logarithm of the odds
- Lod score is the log of the odds in favour of finding the observed combination of alleles at the loci under study, if they are linked at a given distance.
- The Lod score is a statistical method that tests genetic marker data in human families to determine whether two loci are linked.
- A Lod score of +3 or more at a recombination distance of less than 50cM between 2 loci is considered strong evidence of linkage (1000 : 1 odds for linkage)
- A Lod score of –2 or less is strong evidence of no linkage (100 : 1 odds against linkage)

Detection of linked Loci by Pedigree Analysis

Linkage relationships are most easily determined for X-linked genes because all genes that follow an X-linked inheritance pattern are obviously on the same chromosome. Determining linkage for autosomal genes is much more difficult because there are 22 pairs of autosomes. Sometimes, however, a pedigree following the inheritance of two autosomal traits shows clear evidence for linkage.

The human eye sees by light stimulating the retina which is made up of Rods and Cones. The peripherally located rods give us our night vision while the cones located in the center of the retina let us perceive color during daylight conditions. Cones contain a light sensitive pigment sensitive over a range of wavelengths (approximately 400 to 700 nm). Genes code specific instructions for these pigments, and if the codes are wrong, then the wrong pigments will be produced, resulting in a colour deficiency. People with normal cones and light sensitive pigment (trichromasy) are able to see all the different colors and subtle mixtures of them by using cones sensitive to one of three wavelengths of light – red, green, and blue. Protanomaly is red-weak, deuteranomaly is green-weak. A protanope and a Deuteranope can be severely colour deficient. Figure 17.2 gives the variations in colour-blind individuals with their colour deficiencies. Colour blindness chart (Ishihara chart) is used to test such individuals by Ishihara Colour Vision test which is named after a Japanese Optholmologist Shinobu Ishihara (1873-1963). Pedigree testing shows the linkage and inheritance for colour-blind individuals within the family.

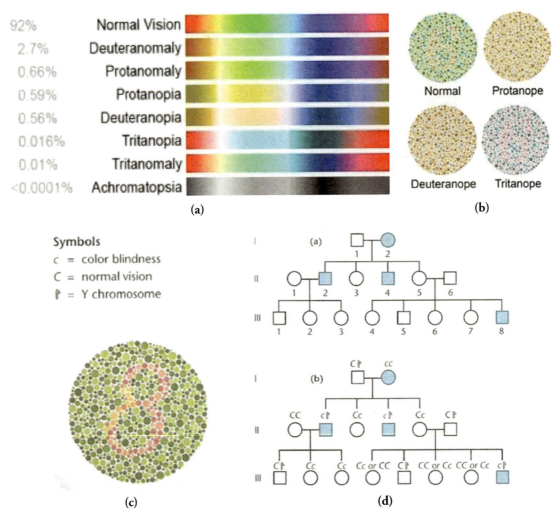

Figure: 17.2 (a, b) Colour charts show how different colour-blind people see compared to normal (c) A human pedigree of X-linked colour blindness trait. (d) The most probable genotypes of each individual in the pedigree. The photograph is of an Ishihara colour blindness chart which tests for red-green colour blindness. Red-green colour blind individuals see a '3' rather than an '8' seen by normal colour vision individuals.

The Human Gene Map

Somatic cell hybridisation techniques have provided a major impetus for mapping human genes. However, more recent molecular techniques have greatly accelerated the process of human gene mapping. The Human Genome Project (HGP) has its primary goal as the construction of maps for each human chromosome at increasingly finer resolutions. The strategy for this international coordinated project has two parts.

1. Dividing the chromosomes into segments that can be propagated and characterized.
2. Mapping these segments so that they correspond to their position on specific chromosomes.

Once the mapping is accomplished, the next step will be to sequence the DNA in each segment. The ultimate goal of the several research laboratories involved in HGP is to identify approximately 100,000 human genes and to sequence each one of them. This is an enormous undertaking considering that humans have about 3 billion DNA base pairs. More details on HGP are given in chapter 23.

The rapidly developing map of the human genome describes the location and sequence of genes and molecular markers and the spacing between them on each chromosome. These maps are being constructed at various levels. The coarsest level of resolution is the genetic linkage map, which consists of the location and sequence of genes and DNA markers. More refined physical genetic maps describe the chemical characteristics of the DNA molecule itself at each chromosomal location.

At this time, approximately 17,000 human genes have been identified, and about 80 percent of these have actually been mapped to specific chromosomal locations. There is clearly a very long way to go. The genes that have been identified are involved primarily in some kind of genetic disorder or disease state. We are just beginning to identify loci that influence normal, non disease types of variation, such as height, weight, skin pigmentation, hair colour, and disease resistance/susceptibility etc.

Gene Mapping

Gene mapping is done at two levels. One, chromosomal mapping that involves techniques to assign a gene or DNA sequence to a specific chromosome or a particular region of the chromosome. The other, the DNA mapping which involves analysis for mapping at DNA level, the detailed structures of the gene at molecular level is given in Figure 17.3.

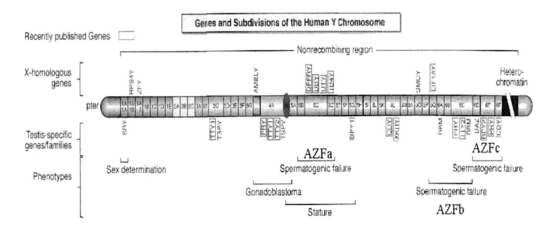

Figure 17.3: Functional map of the Y chromosome (Courtesy: Lahn and Page, 1997, Science 278: 675)

CHROMOSOME MAPPING

The following direct and indirect methods are used for chromosomal mapping:

Family Studies and Linkage

Initially, the first indirect method of mapping of chromosomes for various genes was based on available family studies in large pedigrees. X-linked traits could be mapped on the X chromosome because of their unique pattern of inheritance. A few autosomal traits could be mapped on individual chromosomes because of their co-transmission through meiosis with other well known autosomal genes. When family studies show linkage between loci, both the loci must reside on the same chromosome. The frequency of recombination between linked markers gives measurement of genetic distance and can be used to place the two linked loci in a linear order. Selected loci mapped are shown in Figure 17.3.

Genetic Dosage

This is another indirect method of studying the location of genes on specific chromosomes. This is based on the assumption that the amount of protein product specific for a given gene is directly proportional to the number of copies that the gene presents in an individual / cell. For example, a person with trisomy will have increased protein product level whereas a person with deletion will have decreased protein product level. Direct methods of chromosomal mapping are somatic cell hybridisation and in situ hybridisation

Somatic Cell Hybridisation

Somatic cell hybridisation in mouse and human cells under specific conditions and fusing them to form hybrid cells is somatic cell genetics. The mouse and human hybrid cell contains 86 chromosomes; 46 of human and 40 of mouse. These cells are then cloned. The hybrid cells begin to lose some of human chromosomes as they undergo cell division generation after generation.

Eventually, the cells that are left with are a full set of mouse chromosomes and only a single or few human chromosomes. The cells are then karyotyped to determine which human chromosomes remained. These sets of cells are studied to know which chromosome contains which genes. This is done by several methods like study of gene products or use of labelled probe containing DNA of interest using Southern blotting or PCR techniques. At times, translocations occur in which a part of a single human chromosome gets attached to one of the mouse chromosomes. This allows mapping of a gene on a specific segment of a chromosome. Similarly, other structural abnormalities allow more specific chromosomal mapping of a particular gene or DNA sequence.

In situ Hybridisation

Single stranded radio-labelled DNA sequences are incubated under suitable conditions with chromosomes prepared by usual method. The DNA strand hybridises with homologous DNA sequence in the genome. This permits mapping of single copy genes or DNA sequences on the chromosomes by exposure of the preparation to X-ray film. Labeling can also be done by non-radioactivity, i.e., by fluorescent *in situ* hybridisation.

DNA Mapping

Pulsed field electrophoresis, chromosomes jumping or linking and yeast artificial chromosome (YAC) clones allow detailed gene mapping at molecular level.

Pulsed field gel electrophoresis allows construction of physical maps of relatively large stretches of DNA. Chromosome jumping or linking permits mapping of markers which directionally are hundreds of kilobases apart. The YAC clones permit a large segment of genomic DNA to be cloned. This facilitates analysis of major genomic rearrangements.

Positional Cloning

The technique of the cloning of a gene localised to a particular region of chromosome without any prior knowledge of the product of the gene, is known as positional cloning. In this technique, a polymorphic marker, closely linked to the disease gene under consideration, is selected. The technique of proceeding towards the gene is called "chromosome walking". DNA from the marker is used as a probe to pick out partially overlapping segments of DNA from a genomic library. These partially overlapping DNA segments called contigs are used to walk along the chromosome until the disease gene is reached. Because the disease gene can be on either side of the marker, chromosome walking typically proceeds in both directions away from the marker. To determine whether one has reached the gene of interest, the following tests are conducted; cross-species hybridisation, identification of unmethylated CpG islands, linkage analysis in the newly isolated DNA segments as marker, mutation screening in affected individuals and tests of gene expression.

Candidate Genes

Candidate genes are those genes whose known protein product makes them likely candidates for the disease in question. A selective study of these genes helps to hasten the identification and mapping of these genes. Examples are identification of fibrillin gene on chromosome 15 responsible for Marfan syndrome, without exhaustive physical mapping and cloning. In general, the gene hunting process is expedited significantly by candidate genes.

All the techniques mentioned for gene mapping have enabled mapping of a large number of genes which are responsible for major human diseases.

Clinical Applications of Linkage

- Determination of Linkage genotype of an individual at a disease gene locus on the basis of readily identifiable linked marker.
- Determination of linkage pattern of inheritance of specific form of a disease that exhibits genetic heterogeneity.
- Gene mapping by defining the order and recombination distance between loci on chromosome.

Clinical Uses of Linkage

- Pre-natal diagnosis of genetic diseases eg. PKU.
- Carrier detection of autosomal / X-linked recessive diseases eg. DMD.
- Presymptomatic diagnosis of late onset or X-linked dominant diseases eg. Familial Breast Cancer.
- Elucidation of genetic factors in genetically heterogeneous or multifactorial diseases eg. Insulin – dependent diabetes mellitus.

Clinical use of linkage requires information on other family members besides the one whose genotype is being determined.

Importance of Linkage and Gene Mapping

- Anatomy of human genome is unveiled.
- To develop strategies for gene therapies.
- Heterogeneity and segregation of various genetic diseases in humans is possible.

18 Mitochondrial Genetics

CHAPTER

Apart from the hundreds of diseases of the nuclear genome, a large number of diseases of mitochondrial origin are common. The mitochondria are small cell organelle and they have their own heredity and often always are extra chromosomal in nature.

Mitochondria are cellular cytoplasmic organelle in which the Kreb's cycle (citric acid or carboxylic acid) and electron transport reactions takes place and are therefore referred to as the bioenergetics and metabolic centers of all eukaryotic organisms including humans. As shown in figure-18.1, mitochondrion has a double membrane structure; the outer and the inner, the latter is folded into *cristae* that projects into the matrix and is rich in proteins. Mitochondrial density and the number of *cristae* per mitochondrion are related to energy demands of each particular cell type and tissue.

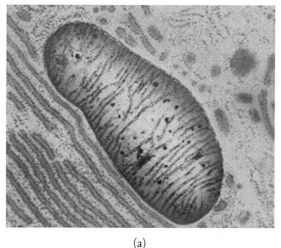
(a)

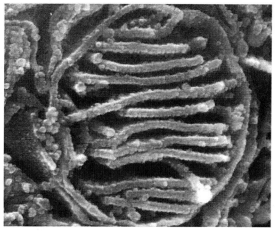
(b)

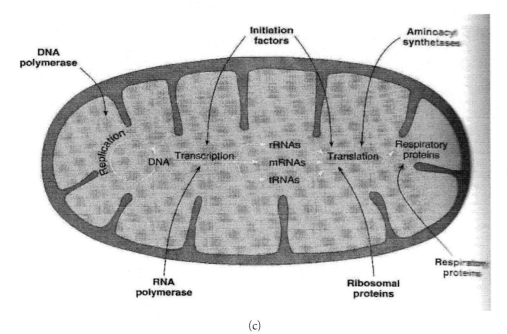

(c)

Figure 18.1: a) Mitochondria, b) Electron microcopy view, c) Gene Products that are essential to mitochondrial function. Those shown entering the Organelle are derived from the cytoplasm and encoded by nuclear genes.

Mitochondrial Genome

Mitochondrial DNA was discovered in 1960 and in short span of time it has been completely sequenced. Each mitochondrion contains 2-10 DNA molecules, the mtDNA is circular small, devoid of histones and contains 16,569 base pairs with few non-coding regions (Fig. 18.2) and is devoid of introns but highly mutable. Further, the first nucleotide of one gene is also the last nucleotide of the preceding gene. Mitochondrial DNA replicates, transcribes and translates their DNA independently of the nuclear DNA. The 24 of 37 genes encode proteins that function in cellular respiration.

The organization and the gene products of the mitochondrial genome has the following features:

a. Consist of unique sequence DNA and is not repetitive.
b. Codes for 13 proteins, required for oxidative respiration, genes for the cytochrome C oxidase complex (subunits1, 2 &3),for cytochrome B and for subunits 6 and 8 of the ATP complex and 7 sub-units for NADH.
c. 22 tRNAs are required for translation.
d. 2 rRNAs (12S and 16S) and 13 polypeptides that form parts of respiratory chain required for translation uses TGA to code for Tryptphan rather than as a terminator codon (Figure 18.2).

Mitochondrial Genetics | 143

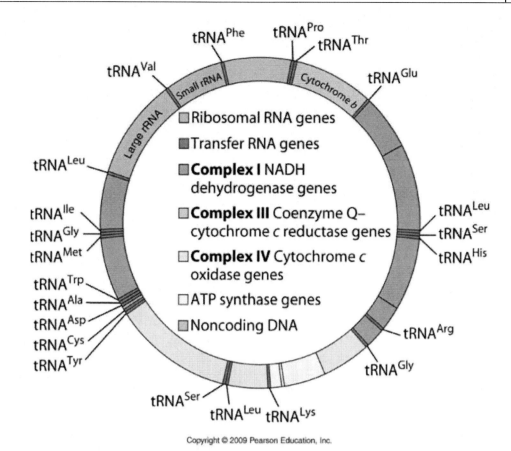

Figure 18.2: Mitochondrial genome organization

Mitochondrial DNA (mtDNA) replication is error-prone and the number of replications is higher and contain little extraneous DNA that fails to code for gene products. Thus, mtDNA seem particularly vulnerable to mutations, since most genetic alterations can potentially result in disruption of either translation or oxidative respiration within the organelle due to absence of DNA repair for two reasons. 1. Mitochondrial DNA does not have the structural protection from mutations provided by histone proteins as in nuclear DNA. 2. The concentration of free O2 radicals generated by cell respiration that accumulates within the organelle enhances the mutation rate of mtDNA.

During fertilisation, a zygote receives a large number of organelles through the egg, so if only one of them contains a mutation, its impact gets diluted because there will be many more mitochondria that will function normally. During early development, cell division disperses the initial population of mitochondria present in the zygote, and in newly formed cells, these organelles reproduce autonomously. Therefore, adults will exhibit cells with a variable mixture of normal and abnormal organelles, because a deleterious mutation newly arise or already be present in the initial population of organelles. This condition is called heteroplasmy.

In order for a human disorder to be attributable to genetically altered mitochondria, several criteria are essential.

1. Maternal Inheritance must exhibit rather than a Mendelian pattern.
2. The disorder should be due to a deficiency in the bioenergetic function of the organelle.
3. A specific mutation that belongs to one of the mitochondrial genes must be documented.

Human Mitochondrial Inheritance

There are over thirty mitochondrial diseases known that trace their dysfunction to mitochondrial pathologies. Diseases caused by mitochondrial pathologies are strictly inherited in a maternal fashion. Most of the diseases involving mutations in mitochondrial genes are usually chronic degenerative disorders affecting organs with, liver and pancreas high energy requirements like the heart, kidney, brain, skeletalmuscles, endocrine glands, eyes, ear, liver and pancreas. Douglas Wallace et. al (1988) showed that Leber's optic atrophy is a cytoplasmically inherited disease. This disease causes progressive blindness of one or both the eyes, with a median age onset of twenty-four years. Apparently, defects in mitochondria are not tolerable in the optic nerve, which has a very great energy demand. The disease also damages the heart muscles.

Deletions and point mutations are two major causes of mitochondrial genetic disorders, while some others recur in different unrelated patients. Mutations/deletions in mitochondria are limited to a single tissue (mitochondrial cytopathy) than germ tissue. The degree of defective mitochondria differs in relation to cell divisions and this in turn to the variability of mitochondrial diseases.

It was determined from pedigree studies that the disease was transmitted only maternally. DNA sequencing of mitochondrial DNAs in affected families result in pinning down the disease to a point mutation, a change of nucleotide 11,778, which is in the gene for NADH dehydrogenase subunit 4. A guanine is changed to an adenine at codon 340, which converts an arginene to a histidine. This is the first human disease traced to mtDNA defect. Since then about 60 diseases have been documented.

Yet another disorder caused by a mutation in the mtDNA is Pearson marrow-pancreas syndrome, characterised by loss of bone-marrow cells in children and is frequently fatal. It is caused by a large deletion in the mtDNA. People with the Pearson syndrome almost never had affected parents; thus the causative deletion probably is spontaneous during development in the child or during oogenesis in the mother. Individuals with the Pearson syndrome actually have a mixture of deleted and normal mtDNA, showing mitochondrial heteroplasmy. Individuals who are homoplasmic for the deleted mtDNA of Pearson syndrome have not been observed probably because the patients die early in their development. Table 18 summarises diseases of mitochondrial origin.

A new technique called *ooplasmic transfer* also called cytoplasmic transfer can enable a woman to avoid transmitting a mitochondrial disorder to children. Mitochondria from a healthy woman are injected into an oocyte of an infertile woman. The bolstered oocyte is fertilized in the lab by a partner sperm and the zygote is implanted in the uterus. Using this technique, children free from mitochondrial diseases have been born.

Table 18: Summary of some important diseases of mitochondrial origin

S.No.	Disorders	Symptoms	Mutation	Inheritance
1.	Leber's hereditary optic neuropathy (Leber's optic atrophy) (LHON)	Acute visual loss by 27years and other neurological symptoms, sudden bilateral blindness, affects heart muscles hence ECG.	Four Point mutation at position 11778 in NDH dehydrogenase gene complex.	Maternal or may be sporadic
2.	Myoclonic epilepsy and ragged muscle fibre disease (MERRF)	Myoclonic epilepsy with neurological symptoms and ragged red fibres in skeletal muscle, deafness, dementia and epileptic seizures.	Point mutation in tRNA lysine gene.	Sporodic occasionally maternal
3.	Kaerns-Sayre syndrome (KSS)	Progressive external ophthamoplegia, pigmentary retinopathy, hearing loss, heart block, ataxia, muscle weakness muscle, (encephalo-myopathy).	Large tandem duplication / deletions, greater the deletion leads to severity of symptoms.	Sporadic
4.	MELAS	Encephalomyopathy, lactic acidosis, stroke-like episodes.	Point mutation in tRNA leucine gene.	Sporadic occasionally maternal
5.	Pearson marrow pancreas failure syndrome(PMPS)	Loss of bone marrow cells in childhood.	Mutation heteroplasmy	Maternal

Mitochodrial data provides a powerful forensic tool used to link suspects to crime, identify war dead and support/challenge historical records. Mitochondrial DNA mini genomes shows more diversity in different populations of Africa than elsewhere suggesting Africa is the centre of origin of man (*Homosapiens*) and traces its origin to hundreds of million years ago.

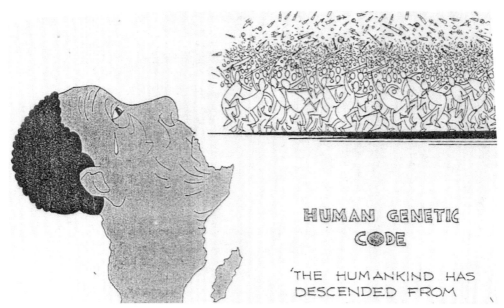

Figure 18.3: Picture Courtesy- "The Week" Magazine, India.

As human beings migrated from one place to another in the past and much more in recent times, the woman carries with her mtDNA, allowing it to diverge in new areas (habitat) (Figure 18.3). By comparing mtDNA variants (haplotypes) based on sequence differences, an evolutionary tree of related populations has been constructed. Based on 147 humans of different geographic region of the world, a phylogenetic tree has been constructed which suggests an ancestral sequence existed in Africa 130,000 to 200,000 years ago dubbed as: "EVE". Mitochondrial DNA can also be studied from ancient biological specimens such as Neanderthals.

CHAPTER 19 Immunogenetics

Immunogenetics is the branch of medical genetics that explores the aspects of human immunity in relation to the genetic make-up of the individual. It deals with the normal immunological pathways and their identifications of genetic variations that results in altered immune responses in health and disease. Immunogenetics helps in understanding the pathogenesis of several autoimmune and infectious diseases. The main concerns of immunogenetics in medicine are, a) defence against infectious disease and tumors, b) Allergic disorders, c) Autoimmune disorders d) organ transplantation and its immune mediated complications and also, e) development of specific, sensitive assays for the diagnosis of disease.

A child is born with an immature, innate and adaptive immune system, which matures and acquires memory as it grows; this eventually declines during old age. It is a known fact that more than 1600 genes are involved in innate and adaptive immune responses. The immune system evolves during a lifetime of exposure to multiple foreign challenges right from childhood(Abbas et al., 2005).

This branch of medical genetics deals with the relationship between the immune system and genetics. It was Edward Jenner (1796), who discovered that cowpox or vaccinia induced protection against human smallpox but this was forgotten for a long time. It took two centuries for the World Health Organization to announce in 1979 that smallpox had been eradicated. The history of immunology and the immune system dates back to the 19th century.

By identifying how blood groups affect the success of a transfusion, Karl Landsteiner was one of the founders of a new science which we now call 'immunogenetics', the field that studies the complex relationships between the immune system, genetics, and the disease. The different blood types evolved in humans in different parts of the world, and the type of blood that a person has is determined by the genes that he/she inherited from parents. The study of blood types and their interactions is just one small part of the scientific field of this immunogenetics, explains why some are susceptible and some are protective to a disease and how organ transplantation can be successfully performed (Figure 19.1).

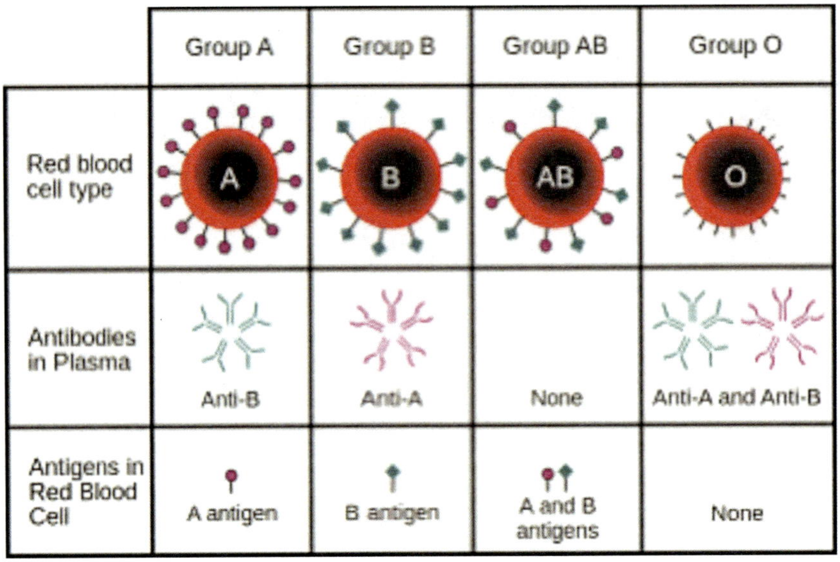

	Group A	Group B	Group AB	Group O
Red blood cell type	A	B	AB	O
Antibodies in Plasma	Anti-B	Anti-A	None	Anti-A and Anti-B
Antigens in Red Blood Cell	A antigen	B antigen	A and B antigens	None

Figure: 19.1 Blood group compatibility for successful blood transfusions.

However, the prevention and early defence of diseases was an essential task for all humans, for the field of medicine and the entire course of human evolution. Fittingly, the first Nobel Prize in immunogenetics was awarded and shared by Dr **Baruj Benacerraf**, **Jean Dausset**, and **George Davis Snell** in 1980 for discovering genetically determined cellular surface structures, which control immunological reactions. The term immunogenetics is based on the combination of two words **immunology** and **genetics**, and defined as "a sub-category of genetics that focuses on the genetic basis of the immune reaction". The term immunogenetics encompasses all processes of an organism, which are controlled and influenced by the genes of the organism, and are, on the other hand, significant with regard to the immunological defence reactions of the organism. The genes of an organism and the transfer of genes from parent to the child in the scope of possible variations are the basis of genetics. Immunology however deals with the biological and biochemical basis for the body's defence against **bacteria**, **viruses**, and **fungi** or any foreign agents like biological toxins and environmental pollutants or failures and malfunctions of these defence mechanisms. Apart from these external effects on the organism, there are also defence reactions regarding the body's own cells, e.g. in the scope of the bodily reactions on cancer and the lacking reaction of a body on healthy cells in the scope of an immune-mediated disease.

During the last 20 years or so, extensive research on various aspects in immunogenetics has been carried out. Both the acceleration of and the decreasing costs for the sequencing of the genes have resulted in a more intensive research of both academic and commercial working groups. Current research topics particularly deal with forecasts on the course of diseases and therapy recommendations due to genetic dispositions and how these dispositions can be affected by agents (gene therapy).

The role of the immune system is to protect against disease or other potentially damaging foreign bodies when it is identified. A variety of threats, including viruses, bacteria and parasites will be distinguished from the body's own healthy tissue when the immune system is functioning properly.

The two types of immune systems encounter the danger at various stages of life and act accordingly.

1. Innate (native) immunity is, **a)** nonspecific and present from birth **b)** encompasses protective factors present in an individual independent of antigenic stimulus (e.g., skin, mucous membranes, sebaceous secretions, pinocytosis, or phagocytosis) and **c)** It is an initial, rapid recognition system for detection of pathogens.
2. Adaptive (acquired) immunity is, **a)** specific **b)** acquired actively by infection or vaccination and **c)** acquired passively by placental transfer or injection of specific antibody. The adaptive immunity is further categorised as, *(i)* Humoral immunity (HI) which is **a)** mediated by proteins termed antibodies and **b)** neutralises microorganisms and toxins and removes antigens in the body fluids by amplifying phagocytosis or lysis by complement, and, *(ii)* Cell-mediated immunity (CMI) which is **a)** mediated mainly by T cytotoxic cells, natural killer (NK) cells, and activated macrophages and **b)** responsible for eradicating microorganisms residing within body cells, as well as the killing of aberrant cells.

Immunity is the ability of an organism to resist infection, while the antigen is any foreign substance like bacteria, virus or cancer cell that evokes immune response which itself is a complex interaction of various cell types and other components. The immune system of an organism can selectively destroy thousands of antigens without harming its own cells. Two major components of this system are the B and T lymphocytes. WBC originating in bone marrow matures in either the bone marrow (B cells) or the thymus gland (T cells). The B cells are responsible for producing specific proteins called Immunoglobulins (Igs) that protect the organism from antigens. These imunoglobulins can coat antigens so that they are readily engulfed by Phagocytes (WBC).

Immune regulation results from a finely tuned network of distinct mechanisms operating throughout life and balancing the need to clear infections and prevent self-aggression. The focus is often on the prognosis regarding the therapy of genetically based autoimmune diseases, which include all diseases caused by an extreme reaction of the immune system against the body's own tissue. By mistake, the immune system recognises the body's own tissue as a foreign object which is to be fought. This can result in serious inflammatory reactions (Figure 19.2) which may permanently damage the respective organs.

Autoimmune diseases include multiple sclerosis, diabetes type-I, rheumatoid arthritis, Crohn's disease etc. Genome, epigenome and RNA sequences of monozygotic twins discordant for multiple sclerosis showed that autoimmune disease is not caused by a genetic variation but the course and the treatability are considerably influenced by genetic dispositions. Patients with Primary Immune Deficiencies (PIDs) have been instrumental to identify and characterise key components and mechanisms that govern development and function of the human immune system. Increasing observations have brought the attention to the fact that hypomorphic mutations in genes that control T and/or B cell development are often associated with immune dysregulation, thus expanding the spectrum of PID phenotypes. Best example is, mutations in genes driving T cell development can lead to defective lymphostromal cross-talk in the thymus and interrupt negative selection of self-reactive

T cells and/or T-regulatory cell function. Likewise, disorders of B cell development may associate with defects of receptor editing of peripheral B cell homeostasis. On the other hand, auto-antibodies can provoke defective immune responses by targeting cytokines.

Applications: Genetic control of immune response and disease susceptibility

Great deal of research has gone into studying the genetic basis of immune responses in the animal and human systems. For example, the immunogenetic analysis of B-cell receptor immunoglobulins (BcR IG) has provided evidence for their role in chronic lymphocytic leukemia (CLL) pathogenesis. The somatic hypermutation load in the rearranged IG heavy-chain (*IGHV*) genes can define two CLL subtypes associated with a different clinical course (Vardi et al., 2014). Those individuals with unmutated *IGHV* genes experience an aggressive clinical course with clonal evolution and resistance to therapy, in turn, leading to a shorter overall survival when compared with patients carrying mutated *IGHV* genes (Hamblin et al., 1999). Solid organ transplantation (SOT) and hematopoietic stem-cell transplantation (HSCT) improved the outcomes of patient management by immunosuppression.

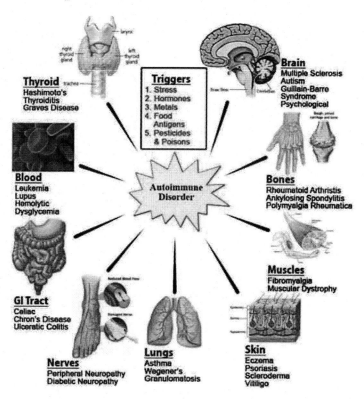

Figure 19.2: Autoimmune disorders

Despite successful organ transplant, long-term graft survival continues to be challenged by rejection mediated by humoral and cellular allo-immune responses against donor human leukocyte antigens (HLA). Prior to organ transplantation, HLA matching is important for selecting compatible donor-recipient pairs to reduce the risk of rejection or GVHD. HLA mismatching promotes graft vs. host disease (GVHD) in hematopoietic stem-cell transplantation (HSCT) (Reed, 2015). The use of next generation, high-throughput sequencing technologies for HLA typing and immune monitoring allows for high resolution HLA matching and helps to overcome the limitations such as incomplete donor typing and ambiguities (Lan and Zhang et al., 2015).

In HIV infected individuals, host genetic variation is estimated to account for about one-fourth of the observed differences. Genome-wide association studies have confirmed that polymorphism within the HLA class I locus is the primary genetic contributor in the host, to determining outcome after infection with HIV (Carrington and Walker, 2012). Diabetes is yet another disease showing worldwide increase and Type I diabetes can be attributed to autoimmune destruction of insulin-producing beta cells in the pancreas. Studies have shown that there are humoral and cellular antibody responses to the islet proteins (Tantawy, 2008). Here again, the HLA genes play a role in the susceptibility to this lifestyle-crippling disorder. HLA system has been found to be associated with various infections. The mechanisms of immune response to infections, based on the genetic susceptibility or resistance due to the HLA genes, as well as the means of resistance to the medications that are influenced by the HLA genes may be the key to future vaccine programs in this direction.

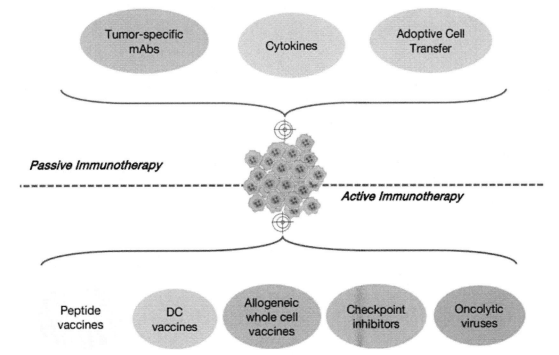

Figure: 19.3 Representation of passive and active immunotherapy for tumor cells

Cancer immunotherapy uses the immune system and its components to mount an anti-tumor response. During the last decade, it has evolved from a promising therapy option to a robust clinical reality. Cancer immunotherapy uses the immune system and its components to mount an anti-tumor response. The two main axes of cancer immunotherapeutics refer to passive and active treatments (Figure 19.3). Passive immunotherapy includes the use of tumor specific monoclonal antibodies (mAbs), cytokines and adoptive cell transfer, whereas active immunotherapy refers to peptide, DC or allogeneic whole cell vaccines, checkpoint inhibitors and oncolytic viruses.

20 Population Genetics
CHAPTER

Population is a group of organisms of the same species living within a prescribed geographical area. Geographically widespread species are often subdivided into distinct breeding groups that live in limited geographic regions. These groups are called sub populations. Humans also may subdivide into local populations. But now, for the most part we exist in global population, except in some isolated tribal populations and island populations. In humans, population genomics typically refers to applying technology in the quest to understand how genes contribute to our health and well-being.

The branch of population genetics is actually a part of evolutionary biology. It deals with the genetic differences occur within and between the populations. It deals with the phenomena as adaptation, speciation and population structure. Some terms to be familiar with include:

- *Gene pool* is defined as the complete genetic information within individuals in a population. It can be described and characterized by statistical properties.
- *Allelic frequency* or gene frequency is the proportion of all alleles at a locus at specified type.
- *Polymorphism* is defined as proportion of genetic loci which exist in more than one allelic form.
- *Heterozygosity* is a proportion of individuals that are heterozygous for alternate alleles.

Genetic variation in population can be measured by checking the heterozygosity of the population or identifying polymorphisms. These genetic variations are helpful in identifying the phenotypic expression of the genes in a population. And also they are helpful in identifying or predicting risk or association of the genes or alleles with diseases.

Population genetics analyze the population by looking at:
- Phenotypic effect:
  Eg; Color, size, and shape
  Colour blindness, Huntington's disease.
- Variations in Protein structure:
  Eg: Blood groups
  Sickle cell anemia, Beta thalassemia.

- Variation in DNA sequences:
    Eg; Alter restriction sites or create restriction sites.

Genetic Diversity

Best example for genetic variation studies in human population is either useful or harmful for certain genetic variations which are more susceptible for disease causation. In recent years a useful genetic variant in human beings was identified which has a protective role for human beings with HIV. As we are aware that most of the humans are susceptible to HIV infection, however, some individuals are resistant to HIV after repeated exposure to the virus. It is due the specific genetic make-up of an individual where a rare allele in homozygous condition codes for CCR5 protein. CCR5 is a cell surface protein and co-receptor for the HIV virus when it binds to cell membrane of macrophages and T cells. The development of this resistance to the virus in some people is due to the deletion of 32bp region in CCR5 gene resulting in dysfunction of the protein. The people who inherit two copies of this 32bp deleted alleles have no functional CCR5 co-receptors thereby develop resistant to HIV infection.

Likewise the evolutionary changes or changes that are happened at population level could be reasons for the protective or susceptible nature and are studied by population geneticists. Evolution is the natural process due to which there is certain behaviour of the alleles in a population as against a background of forces which can cause the change in the allelic frequencies. Population genetics not only deals with the inherited changes occurs in the population in a given point of time but also elucidate the evolutionary aspects.

Hardy-Weinberg Principle:

The relative frequencies of various kinds of genes in a large and randomly mating population tend to remain constant from generation to generation in the absence of evolutionary forces such as mutation, selection, gene flow, genetic drift and inbreeding.

Hardy-Weinberg principle deals with Mendelian genetics in the context of populations that are diploid and sexually reproducing individuals. The following assumptions are:
1. Allelic frequency of the population will not change from generation to generation.
2. If allelic frequencies in a population with two alleles at a locus are p and q, their expected genotypic frequencies are p^2, $2pq$ and q^2. If the population is in Hardy-Weinberg equilibrium this frequency will not change from generation to generation and remains as $p^2 + 2pq + q^2 = 1$

Allelic frequencies are useful in interpreting the patterns of mating, selection of certain alleles and migration between populations. Allelic frequencies are more useful than the genotypic frequencies because, alleles rarely undergo mutation in single generation so they are stable in their transmission from one generation to another generation. In contrast genotypes are not permanent because they undergo meiosis, where segregation and recombination takes place.

Salient features of Hardy-Weinberg Theorem:

- The frequency of gene or genotype in a population remains at an equilibrium generation after generation.
- In a population, mating is completely a random phenomena.
- The equilibrium in genotype and gene frequencies occur in large size populations whereas, in small populations gene frequencies are unpredictable.
- The genotypes in the population reproduce equally and successfully.
- Particular allele will be neither differentially added nor subtracted from the population.

Some of the major factors which affect the genetic equilibrium and induce the variability in population are as follows: (A) Mutations (B) Recombinations during Sexual Reproduction (C) Genetic Drift (D) Gene Migration (Gene Flow) (E) Natural Selection.

Factors affecting Hardy-Weinberg Equilibrium:

Because of many reasons we can apply Hardy - Weinberg principle to a particular population. Some of the reasons may be, mating might not be random, the members of the population carrying different alleles might not have equal chances of surviving and reproducing, the population might be subdivided into partially isolated units, or it might be an mixture of different populations that have come together recently by migration. Deviation from Hardy-Weinberg equilibrium, where the allele or genotype frequencies in a population change over time can be described as Micro-evolution.

(a) **Mutation:** *Increase variation in the gene pool of a species*

When cells replicate, DNA also replicates and is not always a faithful copy of the original; the error is called a mutation. If the mutation occurs in the germ-line it may be passed to the next generation. Mutations may be a single DNA base substitution, deletion, gene duplication and so on. Some mutations, present initially as a single copy in the population, will be lost in genetic drift, but other new mutations will become established in the population, especially if the new mutation has a selective advantage. A point mutation in a functional gene is silent if it occurs in a redundant nucleotide (explained below); otherwise, it results in an amino acid change in a molecule and is then possibly subject to selection. Mutations may be neutral, harmful, or beneficial. Even at the risk of harmful effects, mutations are necessary to increase variation in the population so that natural selection can produce organisms more suited to their environment.

(b) *Genetic drift – A consequence of small population size*

Genetic drift occurs when the distribution of genes in a given generation differs from the distribution in the previous generation. That means genetic drift causes change in gene frequencies of populations. However, it tends to decrease genetic variation within a population and increase between populations. The impact of genetic drift is directly related to population size — the smaller the population, the greater the fluctuations in gene frequencies from one generation to the next and the greater the chance that rare or infrequent genes will be lost from the gene pool.

The two general mechanisms lead to small population sizes are,
- **Genetic bottlenecks** are created by dramatic reduction in population size – endangered species face a genetic bottleneck on a species-wide scale, and suffer lasting effects even if population size later recovers (Figure 20.1).

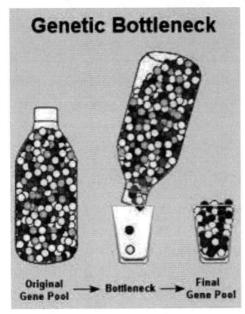

Figure 20.1: Bottle neck effect due to genetic drift

- **Founder effect:** when a new population is established, typically only a few individuals (founders) are involved in colonizing the new area; this is common for islands (Figure 20.2).

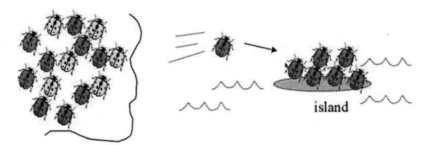

Figure 20.2: Representation of fouder effecr

(c) *Migration – When individuals leave or join a population*
Migrating individuals carry their alleles with them (**gene flow**), usually resulting in changes in allele frequencies. Gene flow tends to decrease genetic variation between populations.

(d) *Non-random mating – Affects more than one locus simultaneously.*
The most common cases of nonrandom mating involve mating between individuals of similar genotypes, either by choice or location. Consanguineous mating or Inbreeding (mating between

relatives e.g., sibs, cousins, etc.) results in increased homozygosity of alleles that are identical in nature. The coefficient of inbreeding (F) is the probability that two alleles at a randomly chosen locus are identical by descent (IBD). Another way of non- random mating is ***Assortative mating***, where mates are selected by phenotypes. **Positive assortative mating**– selection for the same phenotype; works like inbreeding for the genes governing that phenotype, and for loci closely linked to those genes. **Negative assortative mating** – selection for the opposite phenotype, less common than positive assortive mating, but leads to a decrease in homozygous genotypes for the genes governing the selected phenotype, and for loci closely linked to those genes.

(e) ***Selection – Allele frequency change leads to adaptation to the environment***

Selection operates when a particular gene has a survival advantage, through differential fertility or passes its alleles on to the next generation. Post-reproductive survival differentials are not selected because genes have already been passed to the next generation.

Natural selection: In each generation, the genotypes promoting survival or reproduction in the living environment is more common among individuals. These genotypes are transferred to their offspring's. Alleles that increase survival rate, increased in allelic frequency in generation to generation. Over multiple generations, the individuals within the population are better able to survive and reproduce in the prevailing environment.

Directional selection: In population genetics one allele in its homozygous state (genotype) having a highest fitness is called directional selection.

Balancing selection: In population genetics one allele in its heterozygous state or combination of different alleles (heterozygote) having highest relative fitness is called balancing selection. It is depend on either fitness of alleles or genotypes depend on their environmental condition.

Eg: Heterozygote advantage or overdominance.

In Africa and Middle east, there is sickle-cell anemia mutation (HbS) in which homozygotes die at younger age, but there are reports nearly 10% population has a heterozygote condition. Because of this, in these populations (heterozygotes) are less susceptible to malaria infection and have milder infections than people who are homozygous for the wild-type allele. This indicates heterozygotes are having highest fitness in this population.

These are some aspects of population genetics that reflect on the local populations with respect to the prevailing environment and cultural practices of a place and with specific sequence variants that may define susceptibility or protection from disease.

21 Omics

CHAPTER

The term refers to a field of study in Molecular biology ending in -*omics*, such as genomics, proteomics, transcriptomics and metabolomics, etc. The suffix **-ome** is used to address the study such as the genome, transcriptome, proteome or metabolome etc. The suffix -*ome* is commonly and universally used in molecular biology refers to a ***totality*** of some sort; similarly -**omics** has now come to refer generally to the study of large, comprehensive biological data sets. It is the collective characterization of biological molecules of an organism or system, regarding their structure, functional dynamics, and interaction with other molecules. It includes study of genomics, transcriptomics, proteomics, epigenomics, nutritional genomics, metabolomics, pharmacogenomics and the more recent addition of personalized genomics which uses mass sequencing information for personal diagnostics and treatment. All these studies of 'omics' have integrated in themselves, bioinformatics to roll out effective understanding and application of the outcome of these areas (Figure 21.1).

With the advent of the genomics era, scientists have had access to mass analysis and data of genetic changes that are related to nearly every human disease. Simple single gene disorders to more complex diseases have seen the role of multiple genetic factors along with the environment to bring about a disorderly change which can now be targeted therapeutically using the various diagnostic approaches that modern research has made possible. The end point of all these studies is the profound difference that has been made to tailor making therapies to restore individual health, which is a part of pharmacogenomics studies. The importance of diet and lifestyle of an individual has become evident with areas like metabolomics coming of age. Nutrigenomics defines the effects of dietary nutrients and other food components on gene expression and its regulation. Individual nutritional requirements are evaluated based on the genetic makeup of the person (personalized diet) and an association between diets and chronic to complex diseases is worked out in order to understand the role of nutrition in disease etiology. This systematic strategy may then help eradicate the triggers to certain pathological pathways. Proteomics is anyway integrated into these studies for a crisp understanding and application of the findings of nutrigenomics or metabolomics. Proteomics runs parallel to genomics in characterizing which tissues have a certain expression pattern given the same genetic make-up, and how they contribute in normal homeostasis and disease in a certain organ system.

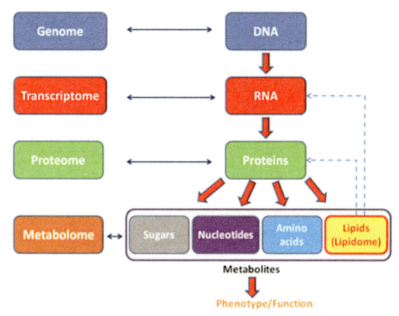

Figure 21.1: Integrated relationship of Genome, Transcriptome, Proteome, and Metabolome

Genomics

It is an interdisciplinary field of biology that focuses on the structure, function, mapping, evolution and editing of genomes by involving f the technology of high throughput molecular biology to many problems, like DNA sequencing of whole genome, expression profiling to find out all the genes that are active in a cell/tissue at a specific time. Further, bioinformatics focuses to assemble and analyze the function and structure of entire genomes and population genetics doing large scale genetic studies on many organisms (more often people) to discover links between the genes and their effects. For easier understanding, a genome is an organism's complete set of DNA, including all of its genes. Therefore, genomics aims at the collective characterization and quantification of all organism's genes, their interrelations and influence on the organism.

Advances in genomics have triggered a revolution in discovery-based research and systems biology to facilitate understanding of even the most complex biological systems such as the brain. This also includes studies of intragenomic (within the genome) phenomena such as epistasis (effect of one gene on another), pleiotropy (one gene affecting more than one trait and other interactions and alleles within the genome. Genomic information offers new therapies and diagnostic methods for the treatment of many diseases. Following are the several applications of the genomics that the current research is focused on paved to ease therapeutic targets to several diseases.

Functional Genomics

Functional genomics makes use of the vast wealth of data produced by genomic projects (such as genome sequencing projects) to describe gene (and protein) functions of all genes, their interactions and gene products. This also focuses on the dynamic aspects such as gene transcription, translation, and protein–protein interactions.

Functional genomics also attempts to answer questions about the function/s of DNA at the levels of genes, RNA transcripts, and protein products. Important characteristic of functional genomics studies is their genome-wide approach to these questions, involving high-throughput methods. Defining Open reading frames, Gene knock out to probe gene function and DNA arrays enable to determine which genes are transcribed. The genomics revolution has left an indelible impact on human health and plant agrobiotechnology. Mamta et.al. (2016) have discussed how RNA silencing comes into play for crop protection from biotic and *abiotic* stresses. To make things simple, Functional genomics = Genomics + Transcriptomics + Proteomics.

The most important tools involved here are microarrays and bioinformatics. Genome projects are very expensive; hence sharing of information at international level is common by gene chip, microarray and internet data basis.

Structural Genomics

Structural genomics describes the 3-dimensional structure of every protein encoded by a given genome. This genome-based approach permits for a high-throughput method of structure determination by a combination of experimental and modeling approaches with the principal difference that structural genomics attempts to determine the structure of every protein encoded by the genome, rather than focusing on one particular protein. The availability of large numbers of sequenced genomes and previously solved protein structures allow scientists to model protein structure on the structures of previously solved homologs. The field of structural genomics involves taking a large number of approaches to structure determination, including experimental methods using genomic sequences or modeling-based approaches based on sequence or structural homology to a protein of known structure or based on chemical and physical principles for a protein with no homology to any known structure.

Transcriptome

The field of transcriptome refers to the set of all RNA molecules in a cell/population of cells. It is sometimes used to refer to all RNAs / just mRNA, depending on the nature of experiment. It differs from the exome in that it includes only those RNA molecules found in a specified cell population, and usually includes the amount or concentration of each RNA molecule in addition to the molecular identities. Unlike the genome, which is roughly fixed for a given cell line (excluding mutations), the transcriptome can vary with external environmental conditions. Because it includes all mRNA transcripts in the cell, the transcriptome reflects the genes that are being actively expressed at any given time, with the exception of mRNA degradation phenomena such as transcriptional attenuation.

The study of transcriptomics (which includes expression profiling, splice variant analysis etc) examines the expression level of RNAs in a given cell population, often focusing on mRNA, but sometimes including others such as tRNAs, sRNAs. Transcriptomics techniques include DNA microarrays and next-generation sequencing (NGS) technologies called RNA-Seq. Transcription can also be studied at the level of individual cells by single-cell transcriptomics. There are two general methods of inferring transcriptome sequences. One approach maps sequence reads onto a reference genome, either of the organism itself (whose transcriptome is being studied) or of a closely related species. The other approach, *de novo* transcriptome assembly, uses software to infer transcripts directly from short sequence reads. A number of organism-specific transcriptome databases have been constructed and annotated to aid in the identification of genes that are differentially expressed in distinct cell populations.

RNA-seq is emerging as the method of choice for measuring transcriptomes of organisms, though the older technique of DNA microarrays is still used. RNA-seq measures the transcription of a specific gene by converting long RNAs into a library of cDNA fragments. The cDNA fragments are then sequenced using high-throughput sequencing technology and aligned to a reference genome or transcriptome which is then used to create an expression profile of the genes. Transcriptomics is an emerging field in biomarker discovery for use in assessing the safety of drugs or chemical risk assessment and may also be used to infer phylogenetic relationships among individuals. The transcriptome can be seen as a sub-set of the proteome, that is, the entire set of proteins expressed by a genome.

Proteomics

The proteome concept was introduced by Wilkins et al in 1994 also called as the phenome to highly parallel, high-throughput analysis of all the proteins present in a cell, tissue or organism. It is an extension of the genome study at once as using high-throughput, automated analysis to proteins i.e. the complete set of proteins complement of a cell or organism is known as the proteome including separation, characterization and catalogue classification to understand their functions. About 75% of the predicted proteins in multi-cellular organisms have cellular functions. Post-translational modifications to proteins make the Proteome highly complex protein functions. Proteomes are enriched with two cellular pathways such as the alternative splicing of pre-mRNA and the other post-translational modifications of proteins. Proteome technology has evolved and refined considerably since 1990 and it is now practically possible to identify every protein present above a limiting concentration in cell by separating the protein isolation, quantification and identification. The 21st century is genomics/proteomics oriented and has a great future in the years to come.

The question why proteomics is important is, 1) to characterise cells and tissues as the human body contains over 2 million proteins each with different function, 2) drug development, this is because human genome shows so many disease genes and we need to know the 3D structure to find out new personalised drugs that are effective, and 3) identifying biomarkers, proteome is instrumental in discovery of biomarkers that indicate a particular disease and offers effective diagnostic techniques and treatment.

Of late, a new approach is to use a "protein chip" that analyses all the proteins in parallel as gene chip analysis for each protein. Microarray is an array of chemicals in a very small area as test of analytical tool. Most of the DNA arrays have millions of DNA probes are bound to a surface and used to test a sample if the ample contains complementary DNA to any of the probes. These are called DNA chips or Gene chips. The features of Microarrays are: Parallelism, Miniaturization, Multiplexing, Automation and the drawback is high cost and need for a specialized Arraying robot and scanner.

Metabolomics

The metabolome is the complete collection of metabolic pathways in a biological cell, tissue, organ or an organism. Metabolomics means several overlapping things; the link between genotypes and phenotypes that rely on the analysis of many metabolites at the same time. The role of different genes in the metabolic network can be found by knocking out one at a time. Such knock-out studies can find out which gene/s is coordinately expressed and hence may be involved in the related processes. Nuclear Magnetic Resonance (NMR) is commonly used as it can find out the characteristic pattern of a chemical in a mixture without purification or processing resulting in metabolic profiling. Metabolomics data are rich in information and there is increasing interest in re-assessing earlier data under different perspectives.

Pharmacogenomics

Pharmacogenomics deals with how all of the genes (in the genome) can influence responses to drugs. Pharmacogenomics is an exciting new field with far-reaching implications for healthcare. This involves the use of genomics technology to study the genetic differences in how people respond to medical treatment. Many medical treatments work well in some people but not in all; the difference is caused by genetic differences. Pharmacogenomics seeks/helps to find the relevant genes and use that information to find out which people will respond to medicine. The related terms are: pharmacokinetics which the study of known genes that are related to drug function and the genes that are responsible for variation in drug metabolism. A related link is Toxicogenomics, the study and use of gene characteristics for toxic effects. On the other hand, pharmacogenetics refers to how variation in one single gene influences the response to a single drug.

Genomic medicine uses DNA variation to individualise and improve human health. Pharmacogenomics discovery and clinical implementation require the technical ability to accurately measure genotypes—the DNA sequence variation at specific genetic loci or regions. Most germ line DNA variations fall into the class of SNPs, or single base-pair changes that occur with some relative prevalence in the human population. Numerous technologies have been developed to perform genotyping and decipher such information at the DNA level. By combining high throughput data with online tools and databases, we can find promising biomarkers or targets for personalized therapy and future drug development.

Genotype-to-phenotype associations lie at the heart of pharmacogenomics. Pharmacogenomic associations may not be detectable if phenotypes are not carefully defined and measured. Pharmacogenomics tests are based on distinct genetic variants that have well-validated reproducible and significant impact on the drug therapy. Early discoveries in this field are tied to anesthesia, such as cholinesterase deficiency and malignant hyperthermia. Both pharmacogenetics and pharmacogenomics refer to the evaluation of drug effects using nucleic acid markers and technology, the directionalities of their approaches are distinctly different: pharmacogenetics represents the study of differences among a number of individuals with regard to clinical response to a particular drug, whereas pharmacogenomics represents the study of differences among a number of compounds with regard to gene expression response in a single genome.

Epigenomics

Epigenomics is the study of complete set of epigenetic modifications of the genetic material of a cell, known as the epigenome. Epigenetic modifications are reversible modifications on a cell's DNA or histones that affect gene expression without altering the DNA sequence. Two of the most characterized epigenetic modifications are DNA methylation and histone modification. Epigenetic modifications play an important role in gene expression and regulation, and are involved in numerous cellular processes such as in differentiation/development and tumorigenesis. The study of epigenetics on a global level has been made possible only recently through the adaptation of genomic high-throughput assays in differentiation / development and tumorigenesis. Methylomics involves the study of genomic methylation where extensive work has been done in the humans; in plants also, methylomic regulation has been found to be responsible for plant environmental responses like the plant circadian clock and also in inheritance (Sahijram et al, 2016).

Population Genomics

Population genomics is the application of genomic technologies to understand populations of organisms. In humans, population genomics typically refers to applying technology in the quest to understand how genes contribute to our health and well-being.

Phenomics

Phenomics deals with how human genes interact with its environment and offers a unique perspective through which physicians and molecular biologist can understand underlying disease processes. The detection and measurement of large amounts of data that describe a human being (the phenotype) is known as *phenomics*, and the human *metabolic phenotype*, in particular, captures information on both human biochemistry and the effects of the microbiome, and this approach offers new insights into the perturbations caused by diseases or by exposure to external agents—be they air pollution, traces of toxic chemicals in the environment, lifestyle choices, or diet.

The detection and measurement of metabolites, which are the cellular end products, provide a holistic view of how particular treatments and interventions modulate cellular function and output. Phenome researchers explore both at population and patient level to detect metabolic biomarkers of the disease which can be used to inform clinical decision making at the patient level. The study involves sophisticated computational power bridge an important gap to better customize health care solutions for patients. Phenome centers abroad play important role in linking metabolic data with patient-level genomic, proteomic, and image data that serve to optimize the patterns of care and improve patient care and resource utilization.

Metagenomics

Metagenomics is the study of *metagenomes*, i.e., DNA recovered directly from environmental samples. This field is also being referred to as environmental genomics, ecogenomics or community genomics. While additional microbiology and microbial genome sequencing rely up on cultivated clonal cultures, early environmental gene sequencing cloned specific genes (more often the 16S rRNA gene) to produce a profile of diversity in a natural sample. Such work revealed that the vast majority of microbial biodiversity had been missed by cultivation- based methods.

Other - Omes /-Omics areas are briefly mentioned below.

Glycomics – Study involving Carbohydrates, mostly extracellular Polysaccharides and glycoproteins

Lipidomics - Cellular lipids

Kinome - Cellular Kinetics Degradome – Proteases

Phosphoproteome – Phosphoproteins

Interactome – Protein-Protein interaction in cell

Appropriate understanding and manipulating bioinformatic tools to manage and analyze big data has also been incorporated and become essential in current plant genome research. This has led to the improvement in the knowledge of plant biology and for the betterment of economically important plants. Several high throughput platforms like the more advanced pyrosequencing, sequencing-by-synthesis, sequencing-by- ligation, single molecule sequencing are available to provide information for future sequence determination needs (Table 21-A). Sequencing-by-synthesis platform utilizes DNA polymerase to extend many DNA strands in parallel.

The pyrosequencing platform is based on the principle of sequencing-by-synthesis. Sequencing-by-ligation platform uses DNA ligase to create sequential ligation of dye-labeled oligonucleotides. This process enables massively parallel sequencing of clonally amplified DNA fragments. Single molecule sequencer does not require any amplification of DNA fragments prior to sequencing. Public databases such as Phytozome, PlantGDB, EnsembPlants, ChloroplastDB, KEGG, Genomes On-Line Database (GOLD) and the wiki of CoGepedia web page provide additional information on the plant genome. Despite plenty of information available, there remains the challenge of integrating this on a global platform and facilitation the translation (translational genomics) of these finding to the improvement of plant productivity, thus catering to nutritive requirement of the world communities.

Table 21-A: Tools required at post-genomics era

Pre-genomics	Post- Genomics	Tools Required
1. Gene	Genomes	Bioinformatics sequences
2. Transcript	Transcriptome	Microarrays, differential display, AFLP.SAGE, MPSS3, Protein
3. Proteome	Proteome	2 D Gels, 2D-LC, MS.BIA.MS
4. Metabolite	Metabolome	Gas Chromatogrpahy, MS

Forward and Reverse Genetics

Reverse genetics is the type of genetic analysis which starts with a piece of DNA and proceeds to work what that does (Genotype → Phenotype). By contrast, *Forward genetics* starts with the phenotype to what the organism looks like and proceeds to work out what the genetic structure is that makes look that way (Phenotype → Genotype), decoding later the DNA itself.

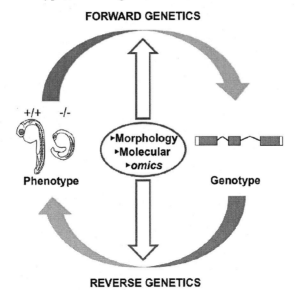

Figure 21-2: Relationship between forward and reverse genetics

Good work of gene cloning includes isolation and characteriszation of the Cystic fibrosis gene are often referred to as Reverse genetics. The illustration above gives a clear picture of how the Forward and Reverse genetics work (Figure 21-2).

Reverse genetics has been used in understanding the genetic structure of range of viruses, including the AIDS virus. In this case DNA structure is known in detail but what it does is not fully known. Mutations are found or occur in DNA and the effect on the phenotype is observed /discovered. This way the function of those bits of gene/s are worked out. The important tools used for reverse genetics are in-vitro mutagenesis and gene disruption (gene-knockout). Discussion on more details is not possible at this level.

22
CHAPTER

Recombinant DNA and Gene Cloning

Recombinant DNA (r-DNA) refers to the creation of a new association between DNA molecules or segments not usually found together naturally. The term r-DNA generally is reserved for new sequence of DNA molecules produced in the genome by joining segments derived from different biological sources

Recombinant DNA technology uses techniques derived from the biochemistry of nucleic acids coupled with genetic methodology originally developed for the study of bacteria and viruses. The basic procedures involve a series of steps. The recombinant DNA technology uses enzymes called restriction endonucleases that cleave DNA at specific recognition sites. The fragments produced are joined with DNA vector segments using the enzyme DNA ligase to form recombinant DNA molecules. Vectors have been constructed from many sources, including bacterial plasmids, viruses, and artificial yeast chromosomes (YAC).

Recombinant DNA molecules are transferred into a host, and cloned copies are produced during host cell replication. A variety of host cells may be used for replication, including yeast, bacteria, cells of higher plants, and mammalian cells in tissue culture. However, the most common host is *E. coli*. Cloned copies of foreign DNA sequences can be recovered, purified, and analysed.

Restriction Enzymes

The cornerstone of recombinant DNA technology is a class of enzymes called restriction endonucleases or restriction enzymes (REs). These enzymes, isolated from bacteria, received their name because they restrict or prevent viral infection by degrading the invading nucleic acid. These restriction enzymes recognize a specific nucleotide sequence and produce a double-stranded break within that sequence. These enzymes were discovered by Arber, Smith, and Nathans in the seventies for which they were awarded Nobel Prize in 1978. Till date these enzymes are categorized into four classes (Type I, II, III, and IV) based on their recognition sequence, subunit composition, cleavage position, and cofactor requirement. Of these, the type- II enzymes are generally used and over 300 such enzymes are known with specific restriction sites which are mostly of prokaryotic origin. In most cases, the nucleotide sequence in the recognition site is **palindromic** (that is, it reads the same in both the directions). Apparently their function is to protect the bacterium and it's DNA from the invasive effects of foreign DNA.

Normally they have 4 or 6 nucleotides. The complementary tails are said to be "sticky" because they circularise. These are called sticky end restriction enzymes. The blunt end type cut on line of symmetry (Figure 22.1).

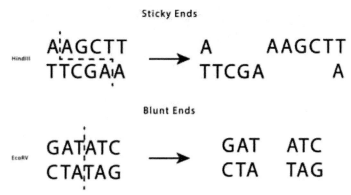

Figure: 22.1 showing the restriction enzyme sites and their fragments

Some restriction enzymes produce DNA fragments with single-stranded complementary tails. For example, one of the first such enzymes discovered was from *E. coli* and was designated as ***Eco*RI**. Some of the REs with their nucleotide sequence and cleavage sites are shown below in table 22.A.

Table 22.A: List of some restriction sites with the restriction enzymes and the organisms they are derived from

Enzyme	Organism	Cleavage site 5' to 3'
Bam III	*Bacillus amyloliquefaciens H*	G.GATTC
Eco RI	*Escherichia coli RY 13*	G. AATTC
Hae III	*Haemophilus aegyptius*	GG.CC
Hind III	*Haemophilus influenzae Rd*	A. AGCTT
Hpa I	*Haemophilus parainfluenzae*	GTT.AAC
Pst I	*Providencia stuartii*	CTGCA.G
Alu I	*Arthrobacter tuteus*	AG. CT
Sma I	*Serratia marcescens*	CCC.GGG
Sal I	*Streptomyces albus G*	G.TCGAC

Vectors

A vector (replicon) is the vehicle carrier of DNA molecule used in the cloning which, through its own independent replication within a host organism, allow production of multiple copies. The incorporation of the foreign or target DNA segment into a vector allows production of large amounts of that sequence. The segments are joined by enzyme *ligase* to other DNA molecules that serve as vectors.

Types of vectors

There are five major types of vectors: plasmids, bacteriophages, cosmids, bacterial and yeast artificial chromosomes (BACs and YACs). The choice of vector in cloning depends on factors, type of restriction enzyme being used and the size of the foreign DNA to be inserted.

- **Plasmids:** Plasmids occur naturally in bacteria, and are inherited as an extra-chromosomal state and consist of a circular duplex of DNA. Two of the original plasmids developed were pSC101 and pBR322, so designated after their originators, Drs Stanley Cohen and Bolivar and Rodriguez. Plasmids possess a limited number of unique restriction sites and carry genes for resistance to particular antibiotics, a characteristic which can be used to identify recombinant clones. Plasmids can incorporate up to 10 kb of 'foreign' DNA.
- **Bacteriophages:** Bacteriophages (phages) are viruses infecting bacteria, the DNA usually being in the form of a linear duplex with overhanging sticky or cohesive ends, the so-called cos sequence. The most extensively studied / utilized is the lambda (l) phage. This phage can incorporate up to 10 kb of 'foreign' DNA. Some bacteriophages, such as P1, have large genomes allowing foreign DNA inserts up to 100 kb.
- **Cosmids:** Cosmids are hybrids between lambda chromosome and plasmids. They contain lambda cos sites and plasmid origins of replication. Cosmids can take inserts up to approximately 50 kb DNA.
- **Bacterial and P1-derived artificial chromosomes**: DNA inserts of eukaryotic DNA often contain repetitive sequences. These are unstable during replication in conventional cloning vectors resulting in alterations of the cloned target DNA. The fertility factor plasmid in E. *coli*, (F-factor) is able to incorporate foreign DNA fragments up to 300 kb, forming *bacterial artificial chromosomes* or BACs.
- **Yeast artificial chromosome:** is a plasmid with centromere and telomeres and permits cloning and isolation of DNA fragments up to 1000 kb long.

Several important restriction enzymes play significant functions. Table 22.B summarises the set of enzymes together with their function that play important role in r-DNA technology.

Table 22.B: Recombinant DNA Enzymes & their functions

Sl. No.	Enzyme	Function
1.	Alkaline phosphatase	Removes phosphate groups
2.	Polynucleotide Kinase	Adds phosphate groups
3.	Terminal Nucleotidyl transferase	Adds entire nucleotide to 3' and DNA
4.	Exonuclease	Removes entire nucleotides from severed end
5.	DNA ligase	Repairs (joins) adjacent nucleotides to make rDNA molecule
6.	DNA polymerase	Catalyses growth of DNA chain to 3' end, breaks DNA down in both directions i.e., Klenow part-breaks at 3' Smaller part-breaks at 5' end
7.	DNAse 1	Nicks DNA between Sugar & PO4
8.	Reverse Transcriptase	Makes DNA strand on RNA template allows pure DNA to be made for any gene.

Replication and Transformation

Vectors can replicate autonomously and thus facilitate the manipulation and identification of the newly created recombinant DNA molecule. The Vector, carrying an inserted DNA segment is transferred to a host cell. Within this cell, the recombinant DNA molecule is replicated, producing copies of the inserted DNA segment known as clones.

The cloned DNA segments can be recovered from the host cell, purified and analysed. Potentially, the cloned DNA can be transcribed, its mRNA translated, and the gene product isolated and studied.

Transformation of the germ line in mammals can also be carried out in several ways. The most common is direct injection of vector DNA into the nucleus of a fertilized egg, which is then transferred to the uterus of a foster mother for development. The vector is usually a modified retrovirus. **Retroviruses** have RNA as their genetic material and code for a reverse transcriptase that converts the retrovirus genome into double-stranded DNA that becomes inserted into the genome in infected cells. Genetically engineered retroviruses containing inserted genes undergo the same process. Organisms that have had new genes inserted into the germ line in this manner are called **transgenic**.

A method of transforming mammals uses embryonic stem cells which are cells present in the blastocyst that give rise to the embryo proper. They can be isolated and then grown and manipulated in culture; mutations in them can be selected or introduced by the use of recombinant DNA vectors. These stem cells can then be injected into the cavity of another blastocyst where they become incorporated into the developing embryo and often participate in forming the germ line. In this way, any mutations introduced into the embryonic stem cells while they are in culture may become incorporated into the germ line of living animals.

DNA Libraries

A set of cloned DNA segments (r-DNA molecules) derived from a single cell/individual is called a library. Cloned libraries can represent the entire genome the DNA from a single chromosome or set of genes of interest. Genome library is constructed to provide a reference source for clones from a specific organism. Ideal genome library contains at least one copy of all sequences represented in the genome. To prepare a library of the human genome using a lamda phage vector, the genome is 3.0×10^6 kb and the average size of cloned inserts I, the vector is 17 kb; therefore a library of about 8.1×10^5 phage would be required to have a 99 probability that any human gene is present in at least one copy. If the vector is pBR322, with an average insert of about kb, several million clones would be needed to contain the library.

Likewise, chromosome specific libraries can be prepared by flow cytometry and cDNA library also can be made by first synthesising cDNA (i.e., complementary DNA).

Cloned libraries have been constructed containing DNA sequences from entire genomes, single chromosomes, or chromosome segments. Researchers use libraries to select probes complementary to all or part of a gene being surveyed.

Detection of Recombinant molecules

When a vector is cleaved by a restriction enzyme and renatured in the presence of many different restriction fragments from a particular organism, many types of molecules result, including for example as a self-joined vector that has not acquired any fragments, a vector containing one or more fragments, and a molecule consisting only of many joined fragments. To facilitate the isolation of a vector containing a particular gene, it is necessary that, (1) the vector does possess an inserted DNA fragment, and (2) the fragment is in fact the DNA segment of interest. Procedures for detecting recombinant vectors involve colony hybridisation.

In using transformation to introduce recombinant plasmids into bacterial cells, the initial goal is to isolate bacteria that contain the plasmid from a mixture of plasmid-free and plasmid-containing cells.

Screening for Particular Recombinants

The procedure of colony hybridization allows detection or the presence of any gene for which DNA or RNA labelled with radioactivity or some other means is available. Colonies to be tested are transferred (lifted) from a solid medium onto a nitrocellulose or nylon filter by gently pressing the filter onto the surface of the solid medium. A part of each colony remains on the agar medium, which constitutes the reference plate. The filter is treated with sodium hydroxide (NaOH), which simultaneously breaks open the cells and denatures the DNA. The filter is then saturated with labelled DNA or RNA, complementary to the gene being sought and the cellular DNA is renatured. The labelled nucleic acid used in the hybridisation is called the probe. After washing to remove unbound probe, the positions of the bound probe identify the desired colonies. For example, with radioactively labelled probe, the desired colonies are located by means of autoradiography. A similar assay is done with phage vectors, but in this case plaques are lifted onto the filters.

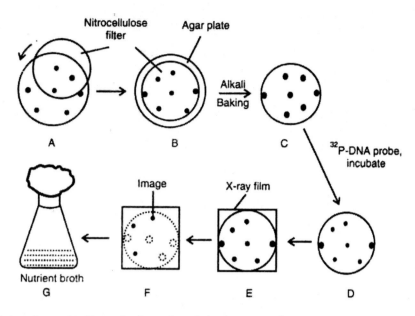

Figure 22.2 Series of steps (A-G) involved in colony hybridization technique

If transformed cells can synthesize the protein product of a cloned gene or cDNA, immunological techniques may allow the protein-producing colony to be identified. In one method, the colonies are transferred as in colony hybridization, and the transferred copies are exposed to a labeled antibody directed against the particular protein (Figure 22.2). Colonies to which the antibody adheres are those containing the gene of interest.

The great value of r-DNA technology is that large quantities of the cloned DNA can be obtained for use in DNA sequencing and other applications. In some cases, it is possible to obtain large quantities of a particular DNA sequence without cloning. The method developed in 1987 is called the **polymerase chain reaction (PCR),** and uses DNA polymerase and short, synthetic oligonucleotides, usually about twenty nucleotides in length, that are complementary in sequence to the ends of any DNA fragment of interest. Starting with a mixture containing as little as one molecule of the fragment of interest, repeated rounds of DNA replication increases the number of molecules exponentially. For example, starting with a single molecule, thirty rounds of DNA replication will result in 2^{30} = 10^9 molecules. This number of molecules of the amplified fragment is so much greater than that of the other unamplified molecules in the original mixture that the amplified DNA can often be used without further purification for DNA sequencing, as probe DNA in hybridisations, or even for cloning.

The oligonucleotides are called **primer** sequences because they anneal to the ends of the sequence to be amplified and are used as primers for chain elongation by DNA polymerase. In the first cycle of PCR amplification, the DNA is denatured to separate the strands and then renatured in the presence of a vast excess of the primer oligonucleotides. Then DNA polymerase is added, and elongation of the primers produces double-stranded molecules; the first cycle in PCR produces two copies of each molecule containing sequences complementary to the primers. The second cycle of PCR is similar to the first. The DNA is denatured and renatured in the presence of an excess of primer oligonucleotides, and DNA polymerase elongates the primers; after this cycle there are four copies of each molecule in the original mixture. The steps of denaturation, renaturation, and replication are usually repeated from twenty to thirty times, and, in each cycle, the number of molecules of the amplified sequence is doubled. The theoretical result of thirty rounds of amplification is 230 copies of the DNA sequence of interest.

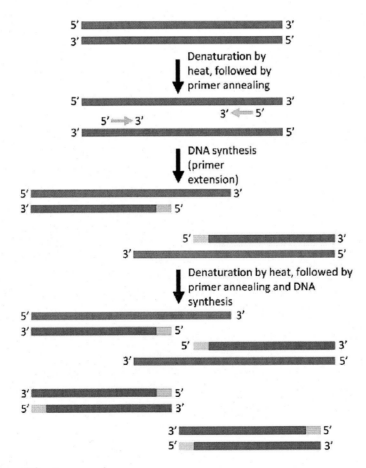

Figure 22.3: PCR amplification procedure

The primers are designed to anneal to opposite DNA strands at the extreme ends of the region to be amplified. The primers are oriented with their 3' ends facing the sequence to be amplified, so that, in DNA synthesis, the primers grow toward each other but along opposite template strands. In this way, each newly synthesized strand terminates in a sequence that can anneal with the complementary primer and so can be used for further amplification.

PCR amplification is very useful in producing large quantities of a specific DNA sequence without the need for cloning.

Application of recombinant DNA technology

1. It gives us a rational approach to the understanding of molecular basis of numerous diseases, e.g. Sickle cell disease, familial hypercholesterolemia, thalassaemias, cystic fibrosis and Huntington's chorea, etc.
2. Proteins can be produced for diagnostic tests, e.g. AIDS test.
3. Gene therapy for Sickle cell disease, thalassaemias cancers.

Table 22.C: Proteins Produced Biosynthetically Using DNA Technology.

Protein	Disease
Insulin	Insulin dependent diabetes mellitus
Growth hormone	Short stature due to growth hormone deficiency
Factor VIII	Haemophilia A
Factor IX	Haemophilia B
Interferon	Infections, cancer
Antitrypsin	Emphysema due to a-antitrypsin deficiency
Somatostatin	Excess growth
Vaccines	Hepatitis B, malaria and other tropical diseases

Cloned DNA segments are used in a variety of applications, including gene mapping, disease prenatal diagnosis, and forensic analysis. In addition, cloned human genes inserted into bacterial hosts are used for the commercial production of human gene products for therapeutic treatment of a range of disorders (see table 22.C).

The correction of human genetic defects may be possible using retroviruses. Some of the viral genes can be removed from the retroviral genome to create a vector capable of transferring human structural genes into human target tissues, where the human genes become activated. Thus r-DNA technology plays increasing and essential role in human genetic engineering.

CHAPTER 23: The Human Genome Project

Victor Mckusick (1969) the famous American Human Geneticist and one of the founding fathers of Modern Medical Genetics is credited with the concept of human genome. The human genome, i.e. 22 autosomes and XY sex chromosomes that carry all the hereditary information from one generation to the next, was approved by the U.S. Congress in 1988 as major International research project for a 15-year period (1991-2005) costing over 2 billion U.S. dollars per annum. The project is a sequel to modern sophisticated molecular, biological and techniques to mention a few, recombinant DNA technology, gene cloning, DNA sequencing by polymerase chain reaction etc. It is important to mention that by 1994, McKusick documented 6678 disorders in his Compendium "Mendelian Inheritance in Man". A total of 4458 autosomal dominant, 1730 autosomal recessive, 412 X chromosome linked, 15 Y linked and 59 mitochondrial diseases based on physical mapping and Giemsa banding technology. Worldwide human genome organization has three centers; for American Researchers in Bethesda Maryland, USA; second for European researchers based in London and the third for researchers from Pacific in Tokyo; apart from the reputed private Celera Genomics Company; USA. The co-ordinating agencies are; (1) UNESCO (2) Genome data base (3) Human Genome organization and Human genome diversity project, (4) National Institute of Health and Department of Energy, (5) Medical Research Council, UK, (6) Genethon, France and (7) European Union.

Main objectives of the project

1. To create genetic map at various levels of all the 50,000-1,00,000 genes on 24 chromosomes which provide the blueprint for human life and mapping of 10,000 inherited disorders, better diagnosis, treatment, prevention of human diseases and to gain insight into evolutionary past of human.
2. To develop new DNA technologies (automated genome sequencing together with fluorescent/ radioactive/ labeling/shotgun etc.).
3. To determine the nucleotide sequence (3,000,000 kilo base pairs) of 22 autosomes and XY sex chromosomes.
4. To develop necessary DNA Informatics Technology.

Dr James Watson who shared the Nobel Prize with Francis Crick and Maurice Wilkins in 1962 for the double helix of Deoxyribonucleic acid (DNA) was the first Director of the National Human Genome Research Project, USA and he was succeeded by Dr Francis Collins. The DNA characterise / digitizes the four chemicals; 2 purines (adenine & cytosine) and 2 pyrimidines (thymine and guanine); Adenine with thymine (A=T) and cytosine with guanine (C≡G) are held together by double and triple hydrogen bonds respectively forming 4 types of nucleotides that constitutes the golden coil of life that is universal to all forms of life including man.

Model organisms

The major component of the human genome project is not only mapping of all the genes but their sequencing. It has been shown that the locus 25 is similar to 17th chromosomes of mouse and 11th chromosome of man. In view of its evolutionary, complexity and large size in comparison to other organisms, "model organisms" like phage (165 Kbnucleotoides), *Escherchia coli* (4700 Kb nucleotides), *Haemophilus influenzae* (1.8 million base pair genome), *Saccharomyces cervesisae* (yeast, 14,000 Kb), *Caenorhabtites elegans* (flat worm, 100 Mbp), *Drosophila melanogaster* (fruit fly, 165,000 Kb nucleotides) and *Mus muscularis* (mouse) have been mapped and sequenced, and many more organisms have been mapped and sequenced in recent times.

The technologies so used have enabled to assess comparative and functional analysis of various genes to understand the meaning of human genome. For example, yeast genome has 6000 genes but only 2300 have been identified earlier. In addition, 3700 new genes were identified by sequencing project; however, only 2300 genes share significant sequence homology with any known genes from other organisms i.e. they are "novel genes" whose functions are still unknown. Mapping of the human homologous of these genes identified from these and other model organisms listed above provide new "candidate genes" for the study of various inherited diseases as also their expression in Gene Therapy, a prescription already gaining momentum in USA and other advanced countries.

HGP Achievements

The HGP is a "factory style" data creation and management and relies on extensive resources, therefore international in scope. It involves coordination, efficient collaboration of over 50,000 researchers in over 50 high throughput labs in the world over a 15-year period involving the use of 300 automatic robotic gene sequencer equipments. The working draft of human genome sequence was released on 26th June, 2000. This is a landmark achievement in the history of mankind and science but also a major technological and intellectual milestone of the 21st century. The draft allows the researchers to delve deeper into the causes of diseases and allow them to develop better treatment and preventive measures.

The human genome is the book of life like the Encyclopaedia with many volumes, i.e. has 24 volumes corresponding to 24 chromosomes (21 autosomes and 2 sex chromosomes). Table 23.A shows the profile of human chromosomes with some important diseases they carry from the outcome of HGP. The data has shown that human genome has 95% of junk DNA i.e. repeat DNA sequences and only 5% DNA is functional and carry about 40,000 genes of which 10,000 genes are carriers of genetic disorders. The human genome DNA per haploid cell measure 5 feet long and only 20 microns wide. To date 95% genome has been mapped with 95% accuracy. It is interesting to note that the human genome is not unique to an individual but represents a spectrum of world population since 150 humans gave their DNA as research material. More information is expected to provide insight on human diversity i.e. how the people across the world irrespective of religion, race and the geographic barriers are one and same as species, *Homo sapiens*. The composite sequence from many sources is generic and represents the human kind against which comparison is possible.

Development of DNA informatics is sufficiently powerful algorithms and collection, software for efficient storage and effectively communicating the data resulting from the project from various International research centers. The rapid dissemination of the information has been effectively met by the establishment of large number of electronic databases available on the World Wide Websites (WWW) on the internet. The online information of the project is available at National centre for human genome research (Figure 23.1). It is expected that DNA Chip Technology will revolutionise the ability to produce human genome sequence data. Maryland, a private genome company has contributed significantly to the growth of human genome project. Mouse Genome and flat worm genome databases are also available on Internet for comparison (Table 23.B).

Future Perspectives/Challenges

The human genome project which was completed will facilitate on short term basis in better diagnosis and genetic counselling for families with a genetic disease or diseases; on long term basis will provide improved understanding of how genes are expressed, will enable us to develop new strategies for prevention and better treatment of disease or diseases (Table 23.C).

The human genome project is a gold mine of genetic information, largest and costliest international research project ever undertaken in biomedical sciences and is much more epic than the Apollo mission not only in its complexity but the benefits that are likely to accrue to mankind.

The project is expected to revolutionize medical and dental sciences for the 21st century and likely to offer medical/ dental practitioners with predictive medicine, preventive strategies, gene therapy and even molecular surgery. In not too distant future, the data on human genome project would herald a new era, where man will decide his own fate than gene deciding his fate. If this happens, it would create ethical and legal issues related to privacy, confidentially, discrimination in society, individual freedom and social responsibility arising from the knowledge gained through this project. The human genome project has already resulted in the development of patents as early as 1998 and when completed by 2003, offered medicare for 21st century, henceforth, Tomorrow's drug will be "Genomic Medicine".

Dr N. Dexter (2001) Director of Wellcome trust, UK predicts that the human genome project sequence will become one of the most valuable maps in our history. He stated that, Maps are a timeless resource and the same can be said of HGP, it will guide researchers for centuries. It offers so many potential uses and is not restricted to one person or to one corporation which is essential for progress in improving mankind's health.

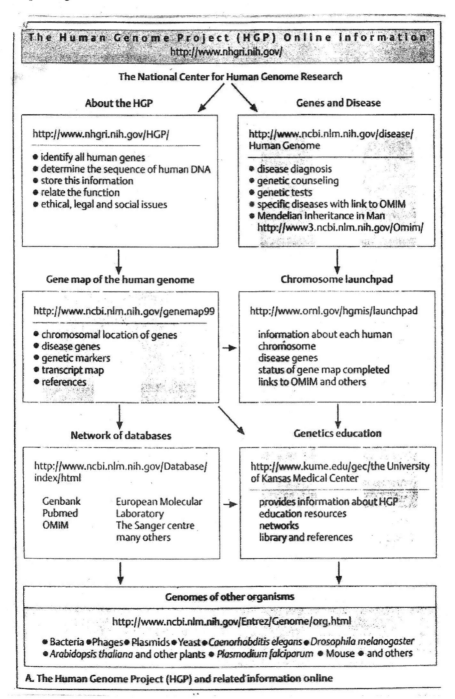

Figure 23.1: Online information on the Human Genome project

Table 23.A: Profile of human chromosomes with some important diseases they carry from the outcome of HG Project

Chromosome 1	i) Gaucher's disease; mutant gene GBA enzyme breaks down certain fats. ii) Polio virus sensitivity PVS. iii) Prostrate disease gene.
Chromosome 2	i) Waardenburg's syndrome; PAX3 mutant gene produced deafness, each eye is of different colour. ii) Synpolydactyly
Chromosome 3	Von Hippel –Lindau disease, VHL mutant gene results in abnormal blood formation.
Chromosome 4	i) Huntington's disease; mutant gene causes dementia. ii) Piebaldism
Chromosome 5	i) Diastrophic dysplasia; mutant gene malformed hands and feet. ii) Colareactal cancer iii) Basal cell carcinoma iv) Acute myclogenousleukaemia v) Salt resistant hypertention
Chromosome 6	i) Spinocerebellar atrophy; SCAI cause withering of cerebellum. ii) Ragweed sensitivity gene RWS. iii) Intelligence gene
Chromosome 7	i) Cyctic fibrosis – mutant gene produce mucous in lungs and pancreas, therefore fatal. ii) Greig's cephalopolysyndactyly iii) Holoprosencephyaly
Chromosome 8	Werner's syndrome; mutant gene causes premature ageing.
Chromosome 9	i) Malignant melanoma; CDKN tumor repressor gene causes skin cancer. ii) Nail patella syndrome NPSI iii) Gorlin syndrome
Chromosome 10	i) Multiple endocrine neoplasia; MEN21 causes tumor of throat and adrenal gland. ii) Epilepsy susceptible gene ESG iii) Hershspring's disease
Chromosome 11	i) Harry RAS Oncogene predisposes to common cancer ii) Insulin gene INS iii) Lactate dehydrogenase A.LDHA iv) Aniridia

Chromosome 12	a) Phenylketonuria; PAH gene causes mental retardation, blocks digestion of common amino acids in food. b) Holt-Oran Syndrome
Chromosome 13	i) Defects in BRCA2 gene raised risk of breast cancer. ii) X-ray sensitivity gene XRS
Chromosome 14	Alzhemeimer disease mutant AD3 gene is linked with the development of plaques in the brain.
Chromosome 15	Marfan's syndrome; FBNI gene weakens connective tissue rupturing blood vessels.
Chromosome 16	i) Polycystic kidney disease; PKDI causes cyst formation and kidney failure. ii) Breast cancer susceptibility BCS iii) Prostate cancer
Chromosome 17	i) Cancer; mutations in P53 gene increases vulnerability of cancer, BRCA1 predisposes to breast cancer. ii) Campomelic dysplasia
Chromosome 18	Pancreatic cancer-damage to DPC4 gene accelerates pancreatic cancer.
Chromosome 19	i) Coronary heart disease; mutant gene for apolipoprotein E-raises blood cholesterol, predisposes to artery blockage. ii) Diabetes mellitus
Chromosome 20	i) Severe combined immuno deficiency (SCID); abnormal deaminase (ADAD) gene destroys immunity. ii) Dominant nocturnal frontal lobe epilepsy DNFLE
Chromosome 21	Lou Gelrig's disease; wasting disease linked with mutant defective superoxide dismutase 1 SOD1 gene.
Chromosome 22	i) DiGeorge syndrome, abnormal DGS gene triggers heart defects and facial changes. ii) Chronic myloidleukaemia CML
Chromosome 23	X-chromosome i) Duchene Muscular Dystrophy (DMD) mutant gene DMD triggers muscle degeneration. ii) Hemophilia gene HEMA iii) Colour blindness deutan CBD iv) Colour blindness proton CBP v) Glucose- 6 phosphate dehydrogenate G6PD vi) Lesch – Nyhan syndrome LNS vii) Hydrocephalus
Chromosome 24	Y-chromosome testis determining / male development and male fertility factor

Table 23.B Internet/websites and clinical databases

On-line Mendelian Inheritance in Man (OMIM) http://www3.ncbi.nlm.nih.gov/ornim/ *On-line access to McKusick's catalogue, an invaluable resource.* Genome Database http://gdbwww.org/ *The human genome database* Human Genome Organization http://hugo.gdb.org/ *Website of the international organization of scientists involved in the global initiative to map and sequence the human genome.* US Dept of Energy Human Genome Program http://www.er.doe.gov/production/oher/hug_top.html *United States Department of Energy's Genome Program site.* Public Human Diseases Menu http://www.hgmp.mrc.ac.uk/Public/diseases.html *Site available to the public for information about inherited human diseases and their support groups.* Science's Human Gene Map http://www.ncbi.nlm.nih.gov./science96/ *A map of the human genome with information about important genes.* Whitehead Institute for Biomedical Research/MIT Center for Genome Research http://www-genome.wi.mit.edu/	Zebrafish Research Databases http://zfish.uoregon.edu/ *Zebrafish genome project information.* Drosophila Virtual Library http://www-leland.stanford.edu/~ger/drosophila.html *D. melanogaster genome project information.* Caenorhabditis Elegans Genetics and Genomics http://eatworms.swmed.edu/genome.shtml *C. elegans genome project information.* Yeast Genome Project http://speedy.mips.biochem.mpg.de/mips/yeast/ Yeast genome project information. **CLINICAL DATABASES** London Dysmorphology Database (LDDB) Winter R, Baraitser M. Oxford Medical Publications, Oxford University Press, Oxford *A diagnostic database which contains a detailed list of clinical features and references for each of the syndrome entries along with an abstract.* Pictures of Standard Syndromes and Undiagnosed Malformations (POSSUM) Bankier A. The Murdoch Institute for Research into Birth Defects, PO Box 1100, Parkville 3052, Melbourne, Australia *A database for the diagnosis of dysmorphic syndromes with description of the syndrome, clinical features, references, photographs and video sequences.*

Human gene map, sequencing and software programs. The Cooperative Human Linkage Center http://www.chlc.org/ *Human gene maps and markers.* The Rockefeller University Genetic Linkage Analysis Resources http://linkage.rockefeller.edu/ *Linkage analysis and marker mapping programs.* Research Program on Ethical, Legal and Social Implications of Human Genome Project http://www.nhgri.nih.gov./About_NHGRI/ Der/ Elsi/index.html *Site about ethical, legal and social implications of the human genome project.* Mouse Genome Databasehttp: / /www. informatics. jax.org.mgd.html *Mouse genome informatics.* Mammalian Genetics Unit & Mouse Genome Centre http://www.mgu.har.mrc.ac.uk/MGU-welcome.html *Mouse genome site.*	The Human Cytogenetic Database (HCDB) Schinzel A. Oxford Medical Publications, Oxford University Press, Oxford *A diagnostic database with features and references on 1200 Chromosomal abnormalities.* London Neurological Database (LNDB). Oxford Medical Publications, Oxford University Press, Oxford *A database for the diagnosis of neurogenetic syndromes or disorders containing an abstract and information about clinical features and references.* Program Listing Abnormalities in Prenatal Ultrasound (Platypus) Benzie R J. (ed) Toikinnoin, Inc., Ottawa, Canada *A reference source demonstrating real time images of 337 fetal anomalies with a diagnostic search facility and information and references on 3500 associated syndromes.*

Table 23.C List of Genetic conditions for Molecular Diagnosis

Condition	Mode	Gene	Symbol	Chromosome	Cloned
Adrenoleukodystrophy	XR		ALD	X	+
Adult polycystic kidney disease	AD		PKD1	16	+
Agammaglobulinemia, X-linked	XR		AGMX2	X	+
α1-Antitiypsin deficiency	AR	αl-Antitrypsin	AAT	14	+
α -Thalassemia	AR	α-Globin	HBA	16	+
Alport syndrome	XD	Collagen IV, α 5-subunit	COL4A5	X	+
Alzheimer disease, familial early onset	AD	Amyloid precursor protein	APP	21	+

Condition	Mode	Gene	Symbol	Chromosome	Cloned
Amyotrophic lateral sclerosis	AD	Superoxide dismutase I	SOD1	21	+
Angelman syndrome	AR		ANCR	15	-
Beckwith-Wiedemann syndrome	AD		BWS	11	-
β-Thalassemia	AR	β-Globin	HBB	11	+
Breast cancer susceptibility	AD		BRCA1	17	-
Charcot-Marie-Tooth disease 1A	AD	Peripheral myelin protein 22	PMP22	17	+
Charcot-Marie-Tooth disease 1B	AD	Myelin protein zero	MPZ	1	+
Chronic granulomatous disease, X-linked	XR	Cytochrome b-245 β subunit	CYBB	X	+
Congenital adrenal hyperplasia	AR	21-Hydroxylase	CAH	6	+
Cystic fibrosis	AR	Cystic fibrosis transmembrane regulator	CFTR	7	+
Dentatorubral-pallidoluysian atrophy	AD		DRPLA	12	+
Duchenne/Becker muscular dystrophy	XR	Dystrophin	DMD	X	+
Fabry disease	XR	α-Galactosidase	GLA	X	+
Familial adenomatous polyposis	AD	APC protein	APC	5	+
Familial hypercholesterolemia	AD	Low density lipoprotein receptor	LDLR	19	+
Fragile X syndrome	XD	Fragile X mental retardation	FRAXA	X	+
Friedrich ataxia	AR		FRDA	9	-
Fructose intolerance, hereditary	AR	Aldolase B	ALDOB	9	+

Condition	Mode	Gene	Symbol	Chromosome	Cloned
Gaucher disease	AR	Glucocerebrosidase	GBA	1	+
Glycerol kinase deficiency	XR	Glycerol kinase	GK	X	+
Hemochromatosis	AR		HFE	6	-
Hemophilia A	XR	Factor VIII	F8C	X	+
Hemophilia B	XR	Factor IX	F9	X	+
Hereditary nonpolyposis colon cancer	AD	mut L Homologue I	MLH1	3	+
Hereditary nonpolyposis colon cancer	AD	mut S homologue 2	NSH2	2	+
Huntington disease	AD	Huntingtin	HD	4	+
Kennedy disease (spinal/bulbar muscular atrophy)	XR	Androgen receptor	AR	X	+
Lesch-Nyhan syndrome	XR	Hypoxanthine phosphoribosyltransferase	HPRT	X	+
Li-Fraumeni syndrome	AD	Tumor suppressor protein p53	TP53	17	+
Malignant hypenhermia	AD	Ryanodine receptor	RYR1	19	+
Marfan syndrome	AD	Fibrillin	FBN	15	+
Medium chain acyl-CoA dehydrogenase deficiency	AR	Medium chain acyl-CoA dehydrogenas	MCAD	1	+
Melanoma susceptibility	AD		MLM	9	-
Menkes disease	XR		MNK	X	+
Multiple endocrine neoplasia I	AD		MEN1	11	-
Multiple endocrine neoplasia 2A	AD	ret oncoprotein	MEN2A	10	+
Myotonic dystrophy	AD	Myotonin protein kinase	DM	19	+
Neiirofibromatosis type 1	AD	Neurofibromin	NF1	17	+
Neurofibromatosis type 2	AD	Merlin, schwannomin	NF2	22	+
Norrie disease	XR		NPD	X	+

Condition	Mode	Gene	Symbol	Chromosome	Cloned
Ornithine transcarbamylase deficiency	XR	Ornithinetranscarbamylase	OTC	X	+
Osteogenesis imperfecta	AD	Collagen I, α1 subunit	COL1A1	17	+
Osteogenesis imperfecta	AD	Collagen I, α2 subunit	COL1A2	7	+
Phenylkelonuria	AR	Phenylalanine hydroxylase	PAH	12	+
Prader-Willi syndrome	AR		PWCR	15	-
Retinoblastoma	AD		RB1	12	+
Sandhoff disease	AR	Hexosaminidase, β ubunit	HEXB	5	+
Sickle cell anemia	AR	β-Globin	HBB	11	+
Spinal cerebellar ataxia type I	AD		SCA1	6	+
Steroid sulfatase deficiency	XR	Steroid sulfatase	STS	X	+
Tay-Sachs disease	AR	Hexosamididase A, a subunit	HEXA	15	+
Tuberous sclerosis	AD		TSC1	9	-
Von Hippel-Lindau disease	AD		VHL	3	+
Werdnig-Hoffmann disease (spinal muscular atrophy)	AR		SMA1	5	-
Williams syndrome	AD	Elastin 1	ELN	7	+
Wilms' tumor type I	AR		WT1	11	+
Wilson disease	AR		WND	13	+

Support Groups

There are support groups for families with many different genetic disorders. The following is intended as a guide and does not include all existing self help groups (Table 23.D). The *Contact a Family Directory of Specific Conditions and Rare Syndromes in Children* contains details of support networks on over 200 disorders and is available from Contact a Family, 170 Tottenham Court Road, London WIP CHA.

In the UK the Genetic Interest Group (GIG) c/o Institute of Molecular Medicine, John Radcliffe Hospital, Oxford co-ordinates the activities of the different societies and lobbies the government and other bodies for improved services.

Table 23.D: Details of the support groups of various diseases

Association for Spina Bifida and Hydrocephalus 42 Park Road Peterborough Cambridge shire PEI 2UQ	Fragile X Society 53 Winchelsea Lane Hastings East Sussex TN35 4LG	UK Thalassaemia Society 107 Nightingale Lane London N8 7Q
The Arthrogryposis Group (TAG) 1 The Oaks Gillingham Dorset SP8 4SW	The Friedreich's Ataxia Group Copse Edge Thursley Road Elstead Godalming Surrey GU8 6DJ	Restricted Growth Associaton 170 Tottenham Court Road London WIP CHA
The British Retinitis Pigmentosa Society Pond House Lillingstone Dayrell Bucks MK18 5AS	The Haemophilia Society 123 Westminster Bridge Road London SEI 7HR	Royal National Institute for the Blind 224 Great Portland Street London WIN 6AA
Brittle Bone Society 122 City Road Dundee DD2 2PW	Huntington's Disease Association 108 Battersea High Street London SW11 3HP	Royal National Institute for the Deaf 105 Gower Street London WCIE 6AH
Child Growth Foundation 2 Mayfield Avenue Chiswick London W4 1 PW	Marfan Association UK 6 Queens Road Farnborough Hams GU14 6DH	Sickle Cell Society 54 Station Road London NW10 4UA
Cleft Lip and Palate Association I Eastwood Gardens Kenton Newcastle upon Tyne NE3 3DQ	Muscular Dystrophy Group of Great Britain 7-11 Prescott Place London SW4 6BS	The Society for Mucopolysaccharide Diseases 55 Hill Avenue Amersham HP6 5BX
The Cystic Fibrosis Trust Alexandra House 5 Blyth Road Bromley Kent BRI 3RS	National Deaf Children's Society 24 Wakefield Road Leeds LS26 0SF	Stillbirths and Neonatal Deaths Society (SANDS) 28 Portland Place London WIN 4DE

Down's Syndrome Association 155 Mitcham Road London SW17 9PG	National Society for Phenylketonuria UK 7 Southfield Close Willen Milton Keynes BucksMK15 9LL	Tuberous Sclerosis Association of Great Britain Little Barnsley Farm Milton Road Catshill Bromsgrove Worcestershire B61 0WQ
Dystrophic Epidermolysis Bullosa Research Association (DEBRA) Debra House 13 Wellington Business Park Duke's Ride Crowthorne Berkshire RG45 6LS	The Neurofibromatosis Association 82 London Road Kingston on Thomas Surrey KT2 6QJ	UK Rett Syndrome Association 29 Carlton Road Friern Barnet London N11 3EX Research Trust for Metabolic Diseases in Children (RTMDC) Golden Gates Lodge Weston Road Crewe Cheshire CWI IXN

1000 genome project

The international 1000 Genomes Project which was launched in 2008 aims to provide the most detailed map of human genetic variation in 1000 genomes. The project was concluded in 2015, by a global effort from 26 populations in Africa, East Asia, Europe, South Asia, and the Americas. Using a combination of low- coverage whole genome sequencing, deep exome sequencing, and dense microarray genotyping, 2054 genomes were reconstructed by the end of the project. It targeted exonic regions and whole genomes, with the goal of identifying rare SNPs and short insertion/deletion (in/del) variants in ethnically diverse populations with MAF (minor allele frequency) of at least 1%. This has revealed over 15 million SNPs, 1 million in/del variants and 20,000 structural variants, most of which were also novel.

The project provided valuable information related to linkage disequilibrium a key concept in GWAS (Genome wide analysis studies) which is essential to be considered a property of SNPs that describes the degree of correlation between them. Also the genetic variation data provided association studies of complex traits and phenotypes including pharmacogenomics phenotype. The project facilitated a complete annotation set for the ~6000 non-coding RNA (ncRNA) and the ~19,000 protein-coding genes in the human genome. Based on these annotations, the number of genetic elements that control immune function turns out to be larger than expected. This allocation of genomic resources has implications for instance, as to how we assess genetic control over the immune system, how we evaluate the immune system's contribution to disease, and what transcriptional products provide the best targets for therapies that modulate the immune system and immune-mediated diseases.

CHAPTER 24
Human Biomolecular Atlas Program

Human Biomolecular Atlas program (HuBMAP) is an ambitious ongoing project to map the human body's individual cells and gets backing from National Institute of Health, USA. This Program aims to describe the "***biochemical milieu*** "and the locations of individual cells in the body's major organs using modern technologies and considered as the '2018 Breakthrough of the Year in Human Genetics'.

The goal of the Human BioMolecular Atlas Program is to develop an open and global platform to map healthy cells in the human body. In humans, the proper functioning of organs and tissues is dependent on the interaction, spatial organization, and specialization of all our cells. Scientists estimate that there are 37 trillion cells in an adult human body, so determining the function and relationship among these cells is a herculean job in itself. Using the latest molecular and cellular biology technologies, HuBMAP researchers are studying the connections that cells have with each other throughout the body. HuBMAP will build the framework necessary to construct the tools, resources, and cell atlases needed to determine how the relationships between cells can affect the health of an individual. The aim is to bridge the gaps in resolution between the current methods of making images of the body, from photography to light microscopy to electron microscopy to biochemistry in addition to software and computational resources as well.

Biomedical scientists have a view of how organs function and a sense of gene activity—when genes turn on and off in specific tissues. Gene activity defines what a cell does, but the organs consist of many different kinds of cells, each with their own special molecular profiles.

In 2016, a group of 90 scientists from around the world launched the Human Cell Atlas (HCA), which aims to catalog how cells operate in different tissues. This effort as of now involves 1500 scientists from 65 countries, with support from many organizations, including the Wellcome Trust and the European Union's Horizons 2020 program and De Aviv Regev, one of the HCA's founding members who is a computational systems biologist at the Broad Institute in Cambridge, Massachusetts, U.S.A.

The American government has commitment to this international grassroots project effort, it is hoped that HuBMAP will have a major role in leadership and building the framework that will help the HCA with about a dozen other projects focused on single cell analyses of specific organs, such as the brain, lungs, kidney, and pretumor and cancerous tissue. Such trials would involve establishing common standards, protocols, and ways of presenting the data. Overall, NIH envisions spending $200 million on HuBMAP over a period of 8 years. To date, NIH has already awarded $54 million over the next 4 years to about 120 researchers.

The researchers will study the cells themselves and determine gene activity information about proteins, DNA modifications, lipids, RNA, and other key molecules using fluorescent microscopy and imaging methods to build 3D maps of cells. Yet another group of researchers will develop the computer tools needed to present these data in a coherent way that enables researchers to explore the atlas; while the third group is developing better technologies for studying these cells. Such development is needed because with single cells there is very small amount of analyzable material.

A national collaboration of scientists has taken the first steps in creating a 3D map of the human body, down to the level of single cells and smaller. In an article in the prestigious journal Nature, the Human Biomolecular Atlas Program (HuBMAP) Consortium charts out its goals for creating an interactive map that scientists can use to navigate through the human body to answer questions about its functions in health and disease.

HuBMAP's tissue-mapping centers will collect and analyze tissues from mostly healthy men and women of different ethnicities and ages. Organs to be sampled include discreet organs such as the kidney, ureter, bladder, lung, breast, small intestine and colon; the blood vessels; and immune-system organs such as the lymphatic tissues, spleen, thymus and lymph nodes. Work on this project is at full swing and it is premature to add further information at the moment (doi:10.1126/science.aaz8281).

25 Genetic Counselling

CHAPTER

Pedigree is a chart which shows the lineage of an organism. It is most commonly used for human, horses, dogs, and other animals which are bred for specific genetic traits. The word pedigree is a corruption of the French *"pied de grue"* or crane's foot, because the typical lines and split lines (each split leading to different offspring of the one parent line) resemble the thin leg and foot of a crane. Pedigree charts are essential for a complete genetic counselling session.

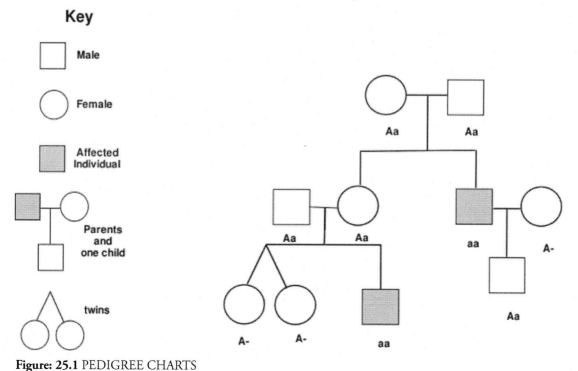

Figure: 25.1 PEDIGREE CHARTS

Genetic counselling is defined as a process in which patients or their relatives at the risk of a genetic disorder are made aware of the consequences of the disorder, its transmission and the ways by which this can be prevented. Genetic counselling is a communicative rather than a directive process and is non judgmental. It includes the following aspects.

1. An accurate diagnosis of the disorder is essential.
2. Advising the patient / the family members with survey of relatives with similar complaints for disease confirmation or in otherwise normal relatives for carrier detection.
3. Management of the disorder either curative (if possible) or supportive.

To enable accurate diagnosis the following three procedures should be followed:

1. **History:** A proper record of the history of the patient is necessary.
    a. This includes both present and relevant past history.
    b. Family history includes sibs and other relatives also. If there is any other person in the family with a similar problem also should be noted.
    c. Obstetric history of the mother includes exposure to teratogens (drugs, X-rays) in pregnancy. History of abortion or still-birth if any should be recorded.
    d. Enquiry should be made about consanguinity, as it increases the risk especially in autosomal recessive disorders.
2. **Pedigree charting:** This offers in a concise manner the state of disorder in a family. Constructing a pedigree with proper interrogation though time consuming, is ultimately rewarding. It forms an in-dispensable step towards counselling. Standard symbols are used in pedigree charting already discussed (Figure25.1).
3. **Estimation of genetic risk depends on the pattern of inheritance of a disorder:** This forms one of the most important aspects of genetic counselling called recurrence risk. To estimate it one requires taking into account the following points:
    a. Mode of inheritance (Mendelian, Chromosomal disorder etc).
    b. Analysis of pedigree/family tree.
    c. Results of various tests such as linkage studies.

In order to arrive at a risk one has to work out the probability. The probability of an outcome is defined as the number or more precisely the proportion of times it occurs in a large series of events. Routinely, the probability is indicated as a proportion / fraction of one. Probability 0.25 / ¼ indicates that, on average the event will be observed on 1 in 4 or 25% of occasions.

Orofacial Genetics and Genetic Counselling:

According to Andrew Poole (1975) genetic counselling is virtually nonexistent in dental practice and this may be because of lack of training, perhaps this is correct. However, many parents would appreciate counselling, especially for dental defects such as dentinogenesis imperfecta, which are not ordinarily dealt with in a general counselling service.

Although most of the bleeding disorders are inherited as per known patterns, genetic counselling probably receives the least attention by those who are involved in treating these diseases. Because of this, families do not have a clear understanding of risks to further offspring, parents carry an unnecessary burden of guilt, marital problems develop because of blame being assigned to a spouse, and the fear of conception disrupts normal marital relationships.

In any genetic disease, it must be stressed that:
1. Genetic counselling is an integral part of patient management.
2. It is the responsibility of the physician or dentist to see that genetic counselling is provided by an appropriate source.
3. Genetic counselling is based on an accurate diagnosis.
4. To help determine the patterns of inheritance a family history in pedigree form should be taken.
5. Other health workers (nurses, social workers, hygienists) should know about the disease and follow through with valid information as they assist the family.
6. Genetic counselling is not decision making for families, but providing the current, correct information on which parents can make decisions which they will not regret.
7. The management of emotional and psychological problems is just as important as the physical and medical problems.
8. Genetic counselling should be initiated early and reinforced several times so the family can be supported and feel as secure as possible about their knowledge of the disease. Appropriate referrals for financial, emotional, sexual and family-planning problems should be made.

From the foregoing, it is apparent that is prerequisite of good family counselling is a thorough family history. This should include not only the genealogy of the particular defect but also a record of all pregnancies regardless of outcome, stillbirths, and all other defects. In addition, a good prenatal history is essential and every effort should be made to follow up on drugs, illnesses, and other problems which the mother experienced during pregnancy. This aspect of the counselling may help to eliminate those clefts which have a "pure" genetic etiology or have a pronounced environmental or teratologic involvement and which will therefore not follow the counselling based on multifactorial inheritance. The following facts should be remembered with respect to cleft lip and cleft palate.

1. An affected female has a greater chance of having an affected offspring than an affected male, although both have 40 times greater risk than the population risk, i.e., 0.001 for Caucasians.
2. The more severe the defect in the parent the greater the risk for an affected offspring. For example, a parent with bilateral cleft of the lip and palate is more likely to have an affected offspring than a parent with a unilateral cleft of the lip. The greatest risk in this sense is of the severely affected female parent.
3. A first degree relative (son, daughter, brother, sister) has the highest risk (40 times the population incidence), second degree (aunt, uncle, niece, nephew) an intermediate risk (7 times the population incidence), and the third degree the least risk (3 times the population incidence). The risk thus

decreases rapidly with decreased degree of relationship as distinct from the single gene inheritance which merely halves. Inbreeding in USA is forbidden by law.
4. The risk for a second child to be affected increases rapidly if one child is already affected. This rises to 4 percent for one affected child (unaffected parents) to 9 percent for two affected children. For an affected parent with one affected child the risk is 17 percent.

It should be also re-emphasized, that recurrence risk is significantly lower than it would be if the condition was single gene inherited. In addition, the risk does not change from child to child in single gene inheritance. This again indicates the need for a good family history to eliminate a single gene inheritance pattern.

Genetic counselling in mitochondrial diseases:

Mitochondrial diseases can be classified into discrete syndromes based on symptoms but the severity of presentation may be variable. They may appear at any age and affect almost any body system, this makes the recognition difficult. While most mtDNA point mutations are maternally inherited, most mtDNA deletions are de novo, occurring either in the mother's oocyte or during embryogenesis. Heteroplasmy is a characteristic feature where there is a mixture of mitochondria within a cell, with some containing mutant DNA and some containing normal DNA. Therefore, genetic counselling is also challenging due to the uncertainties in prognosis.

Other salient points include:
- Some disorders of mitochondrial function are due to nuclear gene mutations. Here, the recurrence risk prediction is fairly straightforward.
- Many disorders caused by mitochondrial mutations are sporadic.
- It is not known whether the degree of heteroplasmy in the mother determines the risk to offspring.
- Severity is very variable and difficult to predict.
- It is difficult to advise asymptomatic relatives who carry the mitochondrial mutation.

For the genetic counselor, it is necessary to determine its mode of inheritance and collect a pedigree including 'soft signs' in all the family members like seizures, general fatigue, gastrointestinal complaints, migraine etc. As of now reliable prenatal testing is not available and treatment options are limited. Newer approaches involving whole exome study have helped in better understanding of patients and care providers can deal with the unsure risks and prognosis that come with the diagnosis of a mitochondrial condition.

Counselling in Autism

Autism is a neuro-developmental, multigenic disorder with a complex genetic etiology, with >1000 genes involved, each influencing to a variable extent, the phenotypic expression or suppression of autistic features. Carriers of common genetic variants associated with autism risk from past studies were mostly found to have issues related to altered brain connectivity. Most people who develop ASD have no reported family history of autism, suggesting that random, rare, and possibly many gene mutations are likely to affect a person's risk. In some cases, autism spectrum disorders may also be associated with various conditions affecting brain development, such as maternal rubella, tuberous sclerosis or post-encephalitic states but the frequency of such findings remains uncertain (Ahuja et al, 2013).Next generation sequencing comes in as a handy clinical tool for identifying molecular changes that may be pathologically associated with the disease. Identifying molecular variants that can be targeted for therapeutic intervention will provide an applicative purpose to studies such as the current one. Therapeutic molecules can be designed to target genetic variants and help alleviate specific and related symptoms in the patient. Appropriate counseling is provided to the family of the proband based on the whole exome or clinical exome based on the testing done in the affected individual.

26
CHAPTER
Gene Therapy

Deliberate alteration of human genome for alleviation of disease is called 'Gene therapy'. Gene therapy uses molecular genetics techniques to treat a disorder by inserting a corrected gene into a patient's cells (bearing the faulty gene) which may be used instead of using drugs or surgery, after the condition appears in the individual. Genetic disorders may however, be amenable to treatment, either symptomatic or potentially curative. Treatment may range from conventional drug or dietary management and surgery to the future possibility of gene therapy/Molecular/genomic medicine.

Since this technology is relatively new, the risks are unpredictable; several medical researchers, institutions, and regulatory agencies are working towards ensuring that gene therapy is well-described before it finds application to human systems. A carrier called the vector is used to deliver the corrected copy of the gene to the patient's target cells. The most common types of vectors are viruses that have been genetically altered to carry normal human DNA. Target cells are initially infected with the vector which then transfers its genetic material containing the therapeutic human gene into the target cell. The target tissue is monitored for the generation of a functional protein product from the therapeutic gene which is theoretically can be said to restore the target cell to a normal state.

The prospect of curing genetic disorder with gene therapy is being investigated and debated. Several experimental strategies have shown that gene transfer is possible. Germ line gene therapy is universally viewed as ethically unacceptable as it affects gonads. All gene therapy strategies to date on humans have been directed at somatic cells only. It has become a promising modality of treatment for deadly cancers. An FDA approved technology, called CAR-T (Chimeric antigen receptor-T cell) cell therapy in the U.S. was the treatment for childhood leukemia from Novartis Pharmaceuticals. A second gene therapy for lymphomas called Yescarta, that acts like a 'living drug', has also been approved by the FDA, for patients on whom two earlier cancer drugs didn't work or had stopped working. Gene therapies for blood cancers are being continually tested and scientists think they may work for solid tumors within several years.

While somatic cell gene therapy is generally viewed as being acceptable as this is seen as similar to existing treatments such as organ transplantation. There are two methods of gene therapy, the viral which uses retrovirus, adenovirus etc and the physical method which employs liposome or oligonucleotides.

Human gene therapy as per guidelines of NIH (USA) is as follows:
1. The gene must be cloned and well characterised i.e. must be available in pure form.
2. An effective method must be available for delivering the gene into derived tissue(s) or cells.
3. The risk of gene therapy to the patient must have been carefully evaluated and shown to be minimal.
4. The disease must not be treatable by any other strategies.
5. Data must be available from preliminary experiments with animal models or human cells and must indicate that the proposed gene therapy should be effective.

The first gene therapy in humans was performed in 1990 on a 4year old girl. She was treated with the transgene for adenosine deaminase deficient-severe combined immunodeficiency disease (ADA-SCID). This is a rare autosomal disease of the immune system. Several patients have since been treated in USA and are school going and receive ADA treatment on regular basis. The somatic cell gene therapy holds great promise with the identification and cloning of several genes that cause serious human diseases. Gene therapy is on the horizon for sufferers of the diseases like PKU, Thalassaemias, Duchenne muscular dystrophy, SCA (spinocerebellar ataxia), Lesch–Nyhan syndrome (defect in protein metabolism), and Hurler syndrome (defect of polysaccharide metabolism). Table 26.A is a summary of various methods of gene therapy for specific diseases.

Current gene therapy involves gene additions i.e. simply adding functional copies of the gene that is defective in the patient to the genome of recipient cells. The inserted gene gets randomly on the chromosome of the host cell. This ideal protocol for gene therapy is to replace the defective gene with a functional one i.e. targeted gene replacement. Table 26.B contains summary of treatment of various genetic disorders.

Ethical issues

1. Somatic gene therapy risks are not different from the risks associated with vaccines or antineoplastic agents. Somatic gene therapies must be subjected to critical assessment of safety and efficacy as any other therapies.
2. Somatic gene therapy is designed to avoid germline transfer/inadvertant germline. Therapy may still be possible. Risk of genetic damage is transmitted to the offspring is not unique to gene therapy. This concern is not different from cancer radio and chemotherapy.
3. Patients with somatic gene therapy still carry genes in gonads; therefore, this is called Euphenics and not Eugenics.
4. Somatic gene therapy has potential risk of

a. Induction of neoplasia within target tissue by action of vector/inactivation of proto-oncogenes.
b. Damage/inactivation of other genes in target cells.
c. Alteration of germ line should not occur because therapeutic intervention is limited to somatic cells only.

Table 26.A: Examples of Various Methods For Treating Genetic Disease

Treatment		Disorder
Enzyme induction by drugs		
Phenobarbitone	:	Congenital non-haemolytic jaundice
Replacement of deficient enzyme/protein		
Blood transfusion	:	SCID due to adenosine deaminase deficiency
Bone marrow transplantation		
Enzyme/protein preparations	:	Mucopolysaccharidoses
Trypsin	:	Trypsinogen deficiency
a1 – Antitrypsin	:	a1 – Antitrypsin deficiency
Cruoprecipitate/factor VIII	:	Haemophilia A
a - Glucosidase	:	Gaucher's disease
Replacement of deficient vitamin or coenzyme		
B_6	:	Homocystinuria
B_{12}	:	Methylmalonicacidaemia
Biotin	:	Proprionicacidaemia
D	:	Vitamin D – resistant rickets
Replacement of deficient product		
Cortisone		Congenital adrenal hyperplasia
Thyroxine		Congenital hypothroidism
Substrate restriction in diet		
Amino acids		
Phenylalanine	:	Phenylketonuria
Leucine, isoleucine, valine	:	Maple syrup urine disease
Carbohydrate: Galactose	:	GalactosemiaFamilial
Lipid: Cholesterol	:	hypercholesterolaemia
Protein	:	Urea cycle disorders

Drug therapy		
Aminocaproic acid	:	Angioneurotic oedema
Dantrolene	:	Malignant hyperthermia
Cholestyramine	:	Familial hypercholesterolaemia
Pancreatic enzymes	:	Cystic fibrosis
Penicillamine	:	Wilson's disease, cystinuria
Drug/dietary avoidance		
Sulphonamides	:	G6PD deficiency
Barbiturates	:	Porphyria
Replacement of diseases tissue		
Kidney transplantation	:	Adult polycystic kidney disease, Fabry's disease
Bone marrow transplantation	:	X-linked SCID, Wiskott – Aldrich syndrome
Removal of diseases tissue		
Colectomy	:	Polyposis coli
Splenectomy	:	Hereditary spherocytosis

The Nobel Prize for Physiology or Medicine in 2012 was jointly awarded to Sir John Gurdon and Shinya Yamanaka for their work on 'Somatic cell reprogramming into embryonic stem (ES)-like cells', demonstrated that mature cells could be made pluripotent by somatic cell nuclear transfer or by transgenes encoding four transcription factors. Meanwhile, currently the FDA looks all set to approve the gene therapy for a rare form of inherited childhood blindness called Leber congenital amaurosis. A replacement form of RPE65 gene is applied locally where it gets copied into the retinal cells. Hundreds of such trials are underway to discover methods and molecules that can be delivered to the human cells to correct or replace defective genes and restore normal tissue functioning.

Stem cells they are unspecialized cells capable of renewing themselves through cell division. More than 30 years ago, in 1981, scientists discovered methods to derive embryonic stem cells from early mouse embryos. Further studies on mouse stem cells in 1998 led to the discovery of a method to derive stem cells from human embryos which were called human embryonic stem cells. Stem cells essentially maybe embryonic stem cells and non-embryonic adult stem cells. In 2006, researchers identified conditions that would allow specialized adult cells to be to assume a stem cell-like role and this new type of stem cell was called induced pluripotent stem cells (iPSCs).

Table 26.B: Genetic and Non-Genetic diseases which can potentially be treated by Gene Therapy

Genetic disorder	Defect
Immune deficiency	Adenosine deaminase deficiency Purine nucleoside phosphorylase deficiency Chronic granulomatous disease
Hyperchloesterolaemia	Low density lipoprotein receptor abnormalities
Hemophilia	Factor VIII deficiency (A) Factor IX deficiency (B)
Gaucher's disease	Glucocerebrosidase deficiency
Mucopolysaccharidosis VII	β- glucuronidase deficiency
Emphysema	α_1 – Antitrypsin deficiency
Cystic fibrosis	CFTR mutations
Phenylketonuria	Phenylalanine hydroxylase deficiency
Urea cycle abnormalities	
Hyperammonaemia	Ornithine transcarbamylase deficiency Argininosuccinate
Citrullinaemia	synthetase deficiency
Muscular dystrophy	Dystrophin mutations
Thalassaemia/sickle cell disease	α - and β globin mutations

In many tissues, stem cells serve as a sort of internal repair system, dividing without limit to replenish other cells. When a stem cell divides, each new cell has the potential to either remain a stem cell or generate another type of cell with a specified function such as a blood cell or brain cell.

At the University of Nevada, Las Vegas (UNLV), the research group consisting of Biomedical sciences professor Karl Kingsley and Advanced education program in orthodontics director James Mah, have discovered that tooth root pulps, especially from the wisdom teeth if extracted before the age of 30 years, could be used to generate both pluripotent and multipotent cells. Most of the wisdom tooth extractions that happen, are healthy and contain viable tooth root pulp that can reproducing cells which have been damaged due to injuries or disease. They have worked on a method of extracting 80percent viable cells by introducing a fracture that breaks the tooth into half, thus improving the harvest and the number of cells available for use. Embryonic stem cells work as pluripotent stem cells, which means they can grow into any cell type while these root pulp derived cells can be pluri- as well as -multi-potent.

Umbilical cord derived stem cells (allogeneic mesenchymal) are being considered for therapy for example in autism where they are more potent than the bone marrow derived cells for instance and there is no rejection risk as the body does not recognize them as foreign.

Stem cells

Stem cells are naturally occurring cells in the body that can divide to make more cells and capable of making other types of cells by a process called differentiation by creating growth factors (hormonal growth factors/ steroids that nurse ailing cells and preventing them from dying cells. Few decades' back stem cells were touted as the next frontier in medicines and indeed stems cells is dream treatment now. As of now the information available deals only with the mammalian stem cells.

There are different classifications of stem cells.

1. **Pluripotent/totipotent**: these cells turn into several other types of cells, and called totipotent that means capable of multiplication.
2. **Embryo/Embryos:** These contain many types of stem cells which may be absent in adult and have different biochemical characteristics. These cells usually determined into three main cells lineages of the body, ectoderm (skin, nerve and brain) and mesoderm (muscle and bone) and endoderm (liver and guts).
3. **Tissue specific stem cells:** These cells in the adults are capable to renew themselves if damaged and called as hematopoietic(blood making) and sometime CD34+ cells as they occur on cell surface as CD34 antigens and are totipotent.
4. **Embryonic carcinoma cells:** These are stem cells derived from teratomas (a benign cancer of the reproductive cells).

Applications

Stem cells are a hot therapeutic topic in therapeutic medicine because in principle stem cells can be used to replace any damaged cell/s in the body, either in brain or liver. Stem-cell therapy promise relief from an array of ailments to treat /prevent a disease or condition from spinal cord injury, stroke and brain, Parkinson's disease, several other neurodegenerative diseases, and also conditions such as diabetes and heart disease, blood-cell formation, pancreatic beta cells, leukemia, regrowing teeth, lymphoma and in orthopedics especially knee and some forms of blindness and vision impairment in degenerative, auto-immune, and inflammatory diseases.

Stem cells have fueled the mushrooming growth of private stem cells clinics clinics/banks market directly to consumers and many hospitals abroad in India provide this facility and people are happy with its benefit. In India, Bharath Stem cells registry based in Delhi (www.bharathstemregistry.org) acts as a platform for coordination and cooperation between the donors and recipients collects donors' stem cells as voluntary services. See more (Email:bharathstemcellregistry@gmail.com).

27 Eugenics
CHAPTER

The term eugenics was introduced by Charles Darwin's cousin Francis Galton in 1883 and refers to as the improvement of a population by selection of only its "best" specimens for breeding; It can also be defined as improvement of the human species by selective breeding. For centuries, selective breeding has been used successfully used in plants and domesticated animals. The best specimens/varieties/breeds were crossed to improve the quality of the stocks. Eugenics attempts to apply the same principle. According to Stern (1960) eugenics is the study of agencies under social control that may improve or impair the hereditary qualities of future generations of man, either physically or mentally. In the late 19th century, Galton and others began to promote this idea of using selective breeding to improve the human species thereby initiating the so called eugenic movement. There are two aspects of the subject.

Positive (progressive) eugenics: seeks to increase the propagation of the most desirable types of people in the population/society. This deals with furthering the increase of alleles which cause desirable phenotypes or at least guarding the decrease of such alleles i.e. euphenics.

Negative (preventive) eugenics: seeks to decrease the propagation of less desirable types of people in the society. The aim of the negative eugenics is to prevent the increase of the presence of alleles which produce undesirable phenotypes.

Eugenic policies became quite popular in Europe and North America during the beginning of the 20th century. Some of the proponents of eugenics were eminent scientists but their advocacy was often based on unconvincing data or on interpretations/extrapolations that went far beyond the facts. The popularity of eugenics was partly due to contemporary social and cultural norms, which included broad acceptance of racism imperialism and social Darwinism.

Eugenics was used to provide scientific support for restrictive immigration policies, laws prohibiting marriage on the basis of race and certain handicaps and laws requiring sterilization of people considered to have serious genetic defects. A perversion of eugenic doctrine was used as a scientific basis for the extermination of Jews and other ethnic minorities by the Nazis during the Second World War.

The current understanding of genetics provides little scientific support for eugenic programs, all of which must entail subjugation of the interests of the individual to the interest of the future society and thus loss of personal freedom. Many scientists began to appreciate the theoretical and eugenic programs, eugenics became totally discredited when it can to be used in Nazi Germany as justification for mass murder. There are two major difficulties in planning eugenic program:

1. The scientific problem of determining which characters are truly heritable and to what extent heredity is contributory to the trait and,
2. The insoluble ethical issues involved in determining who will decide when one traits more desirable than another and how reproductive behavior can be influenced to further eugenic program.

It must be remembered that vast majority of human traits are complex in their inheritance pattern and are influenced by the environmental factors is narrow in scope. Equally important is and unclear, how we might balance individual's personal autonomy, privacy rights with legitimate public health concerns without subordinating the individual to a theoretical societal goal of improving the gene pool a concept not different from the Nazi doctrine of racial hygiene. This write-up is included so that the reader will get an idea of eugenics which is irrelevant in knowledgeable modern society.

CHAPTER 28
Clinical Genetic Services

Genetic disorders place considerable genetic load on population and hence associated with economic burdens not only to the affected people but their families and the community as a whole. Many diseases in adult life have a genetic predisposition like diabetes, cleft–lip/palate, familial cancer and coronary heart diseases. Genetic diseases though rare are largely incurable and often severe. With advance medical technology, there is growing awareness and concern by the people and the doctors of the role of genetics in clinical practice. Genetic counselling covers a wide spectrum of risk, diagnosis and possible preventive cures.

The role of clinical genetic service is to advice the patient/family as to how the disease can be prevented and its implication in the family/society. This service covers several aspects and diagnosis is the first pre-requisite for genetic counselling without a defined diagnosis, appropriate genetic advice may be given to the needy in terms of the mode of inheritance etc. Drawing a pedigree is the best way to record genetic information as per the international norms. Once this is done, estimation of gender risk depends on the pattern of inheritance of the disorder, with emphasis to identify the carrier. Mendelian disorders due to mutant genes carry high risk of recurrence whereas chromosome disorders are at low risk. Interpretation of risk varies depending on severity of the disorder and this aspect needs to be discussed with the doctor vis-à-vis the family.

The risk of curing a disorder, the severity and nature of disorder prenatal diagnosis, its implication on the couple, religious considerations/taboos etc have to be considered.

The psychological basis of diagnosis involving emotional stress affecting the counselling though supplementary is a very vital in decision making and requires sensitive counselling over a period of time. Department of clinical genetics in teaching hospitals are rich in academic and technically trained staff with access to genetic services for patients/families. Diagnostic and genetic counselling is provided by medical genetic counselors those have nursing or other paramedical background; associated labor services are integral in providing clinical genetic service. These provide biochemical, psychological, cytological, cytogenetical, pathological, dermatoglypic and even molecular genetics services. Finally, clinical use of registers is aimed at ascertaining as completely as possible all people at risk of developing/transmitting a particular disorder. A register permits a long term follow up of family history. The following figure 28.1 shows the interaction of services between various groups. Genetic registers are best preserved in computers and can be accessed for incidence and natural course of diseases, effect of counselling and preventive measures etc.

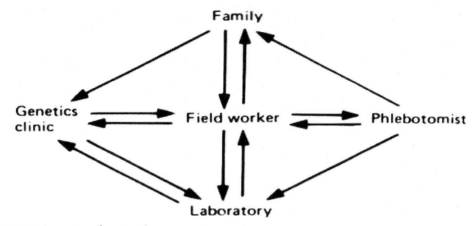

Figure 28.1: Interaction of services between various groups

Reasons for referral to a genetics clinic

- Genetic disease diagnosed, counselling requested.
- Testing carrier state of family members for Mendelian disorders.
- Investigation and diagnosis of possible genetic disease.
- Diagnosis of mental handicap or physical abnormality.
- Diagnosis of malformation in neonates or stillbirth including amniocentesis.
- Genetic investigation of recurrent pregnancy loss.
- Genetic management of high risk pregnancies.
- Interpretation of abnormal prenatal tests.
- Inbreeding etc.

Main users of clinical genetic services

- Pediatricians
- Obstetricians
- Other hospital specialists, psychiatry, dentistry, neurology
- General practitioners
- Community child health services
- Others (self referrals, adoption services)

The following (Table 28.A) are the important constituents of clinical services.

Table: 28.A Organization of Clinical Services

Medical staff	* Consultant clinical geneticists
	* Specialist registrars
	* Clinical assistants /clinical medical officers
Field workers	* Genetic associates (scientific officers /counselors)
	* Specialist health visitors
	* Phlebotomist
Clerical supporting staff	* Computer personal
	* Photographer
	* Medical record assistant
Laboratory services	* Biomechanical tests
	* Cytogenetic tests
	* Molecular genetic testing
	* Pathology test
	* Dermatoglyphic service etc.

CHAPTER 29: Forensic Genetics

Forensic genetics is a branch of forensic medicine which deals with the application of medical knowledge to legal matters. Forensic genetics is not a new field, it existed long before the era of DNA fingerprinting, blood grouping, HLA typing, and other tests of genetic markers in blood were done.

Samples are collected using a sampling kit (either commercial or assembled in the laboratory) and transported to the laboratory under proper conditions. An accurate description of the biological nature of the sample is usually included, and a unique code must be assigned to each collected sample. If the request is part of a legal procedure, not only traceability but also the strict maintenance of the chain of custody (chronological documentation of the evidence) is a key issue. The genetic material is extracted from the samples using an appropriate and validated protocol. However, certain urgent situations (e.g., bio-terrorism) may require the use of methods that were not previously validated. Care must be taken when extracting and storing the genetic material to maintain integrity. Organizations such as WHO and the ICMR (India) are of prime importance as we are currently experiencing in the Covid 19 situation, a pandemic that originated in China and has the world nations seeking for Hydroxychloroquine from India for treatment purpose. Whether this is an act of bio-terrorism as suspected by many countries, remains to be seen. Storage of non-human evidence does not create any specific problem however reproducibility is an issue when dealing with sampling of wildlife or environmental material. The selection of the genetic test depends on the question to be addressed.

Genetic identification is based on polymorphic DNA markers that can provide sufficient discriminatory resolution like Simple Sequence Repeats (SSRs), Short Tandem Repeats (STRs), or microsatellites, and Single Nucleotide Polymorphisms (SNPs). The development of reduced-size STR amplicons (miniSTRs) can provide easy PCR amplification of degraded DNA samples, better estimation of mutation rates and allele frequencies, and construction of allelic ladders for accurate classification of alleles. Alternative methods to PCR include technologies such as nucleic acid sequence-based amplification (NASBA) and loop-mediated isothermal amplification (LAMP). A more advanced post-PCR technique, high-resolution DNA melting (HRM) analysis, which is based on the detection of small differences in amplicon melting (dissociation) curves, was also considered for non-human forensic genetics. Next generation sequencing (NGS) has also revolutionized forensic genetics (Horner et al, 2010). These new technologies provide clear advantages regarding high-throughput due to an extensive multiplexing capacity and parallel sequencing of millions of molecules (Multiple Parallel Sequencing, MPS), allowing a faster and more informative analysis.

The scientific development of forensic genetic genealogy (FGG), which couples genetic analysis with investigation of publicly available genealogy information, has successfully transformed law enforcement investigations by solving more than 50 cases in the United States. However, use of FGG by law enforcement has preceded widespread development of best practices to protect the genetic privacy of private citizens who have voluntarily submitted samples to genealogy databases. Absent best practices, use of FGG could lead to compromised cases, diminished use, or the loss of this new investigative tool. Public support for FGG could be jeopardized and confidence in forensic DNA analysis could be undermined. As the custodian of a national law enforcement DNA database (CODIS), the U.S. Federal Bureau of Investigation (FBI) is looked to by many in the law enforcement and forensic DNA communities for guidance and its efforts often influence the global community. The emergence of FGG suggests that further discussions on privacy, genomics, and the use of genealogy by law enforcement would be beneficial. Accordingly, the FBI seeks to engage the scientific and bioethics communities in such a dialogue.

Use of FGG involves databases and family trees composed of genetic data of private citizens who are not under suspicion for any crimes. When searching crime scene, DNA in these databases, potential perpetrators may be uncovered by identifying their close or distant relatives, and then building family trees that can extend over many generations and may include hundreds to thousands of relatives. To date, this approach is only used if crime scene DNA has not matched genetic profiles in the CODIS database of known offenders. A consensus has emerged that there is no legal prohibition on such use. The question is how it should be done.

Under a recently released interim policy from the U.S. Department of Justice (DOJ), federal investigative agencies may develop internal policies and procedures and can utilize FGG if the case involves an unsolved violent crime (homicide or sex crime) for which a CODIS search resulted in no matches, and for which reasonable investigative leads have been pursued. The DOJ Interim Policy is the first substantial attempt to address "how genetic genealogy should be done." The interim guidance restricts investigative agencies to using only public databases or direct-to-consumer genetic genealogy services that provide clear notice to users and the public that law enforcement may access their sites for investigative or unidentified human remains identification purposes. The forensic DNA community is also working on guidance to address the "how to" question. The Scientific Working Group on DNA Analysis Methods (SWGDAM; swgdam.org), which recommends standards to the FBI for CODIS and issues guidance for the forensic DNA community, formed an interim committee on FGG composed of genealogists, bioethicists, academicians, law enforcement, and forensic scientists, as well as representatives of the European Network of Forensic Science Institutes and the International

Society of Forensic Genetics (the author is co-chair of this committee). This group held an FGG technical symposium for SWGDAM membership and submitted recommendations to SWGDAM leadership that included establishing an FGG Working Group.

http://www.sciencemag.org/about/science-licenses-journal-article-reuse is an article distributed under the terms of the Science Journals Default License.

The Centre for DNA Fingerprinting and diagnostics (CDFD), a government of India undertaking in Hyderabad is one such referral centre for investigations pertaining to forensic cases like paternity testing, investigating crime/accident scene etc.

The human microbiome is starting to be a focus of interest for identification purposes. The rational is to trace human microbiomes on our skin on the surfaces and objects we interact with the potential to supplement the use of human DNA for associating people with evidence and environments. The NGS technologies profoundly improved the ability to detect microorganisms, even when present in low abundance or in degraded or mixture samples, and to differentiate at strain/isolate level, using diagnostic genomic signatures (Budowle et al, 2014) allowed the analysis of microbial evidence to be expanded to cases related with geolocation, body fluid characterization, or postmortem interval estimation. Some biological agents can be used as weapons or threats. The best well-known example is the Amerithrax case in 2001, where letters laden with *Bacillus anthracis* spores were sent through the U.S. Postal Service to several media offices in New York and Florida and to U.S. senators in Washington. In this case, DNA evidence was found in the suspect's laboratory.

While traditional forensic genetics has been oriented towards using human DNA in criminal investigation and civil court cases. Current forensic genetics is progressively incorporating the analysis of non-human genetic material, which can be crucial or the sole type of available evidence, the entire process being revolutionized by the increasing variety of genetic markers, the establishment of faster, and cheaper sequencing technologies and the emergence methods and advanced bioinformatics.

CHAPTER 30: CRISPR / Cas Technology

Over the past several years, gene therapies and cell-based immunotherapies for cancer have become a reality, with several products approved by US and EU regulatory agencies and numerous clinical trials are ongoing. Gene-editing approaches leveraging programmable nucleases, such as clustered regularly interspersed short palindrome repeats (CRISPR)/Cas9, have invigorated work in this area as evidenced by a bolus of high-impact papers and a flood of biotechnology companies seeking to bring edited therapeutics to the market. The potential of targeted gene editing to personalize stem-cell-based therapies for degenerative disease and regenerative medicine is likewise the subject of intense preclinical interest.

CRISPR is a novel gene editing technique which is currently generating a lot of interest globally and discussion in the health field, along with commercial applications in agriculture. The CRISPR is a technique based on bacterial defense mechanisms that use RNA to identify and monitor precise locations in DNA. Specifically, CRISPR consists of two key molecules: Cas9, which is an enzyme that acts as a pair of scissors and able to snip DNA at specific locations; and guide RNA (about 20bp long), which guides Cas9 to the right place on the DNA. Many view gene editing (Figure 30.1) as the new front in genetic technology, potentially offering a cheaper and easier method of wide applications.

The target sequence complementary to the guideRNA is followed by two cytosine nucleotides called a Protospacer Adjacent Motif (PAM) sequence. CRISPR/Cas9 creates specific double strand breaks at the target locus that and trigger DNA repair by constitutive knock-outs through non-homologous end joining and knock-ins through homologous recombination. However, have very low and sometimes barely detectable activity hence the reliability factor of the nuclease designs is still not reliable. It still has non-specific targeting of unintended genomic sequences and this in the human system could have strong impact on the outcome in terms of a therapeutic approach. The targeted alleles often carry additional modifications, such as deletions, partial or multiple integrations of the targeting vector.

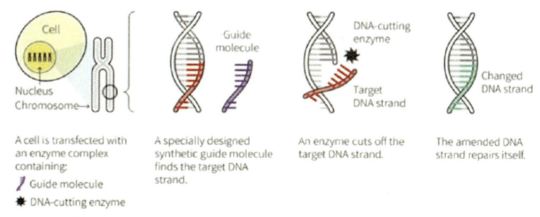

Figure: 30.1 CRISPR/Cas9 Gene editing technique
(Source, Reuters, Nature)

To counter this, it is suggested that we go a step back and apply it to genetically engineered ES cells instead of embryos. Yet another development was a mutant form, Cas9D10A that has only nickase activity. This is very desirable since it cleaves only one DNA strand, and does not activate NHEJ (Non-Homologous End Joining). Instead, when provided with a homologous repair template, DNA repairs are conducted via the high-fidelity homology directed pathway resulting in reduced in/del mutations in the target.

This tool for gene editing is faster since it can be applied directly in the transgenic mice (Figure30.2) or even embryo (Figure 30.3), CRISPR/Cas9 reduces the time required to modify target genes and more economical than traditional embryonic stem cell-based targeting. The idea of gene therapy which has been undergoing setbacks for some time now has finally seen light in the form of Crispr/Cas9 technology. It has boosted various areas of research pertaining to human disease and introducing therapeutic elements or removing disease related segments from our genetic material. With the method offered by CRISPR/Cas9, editing the genetic information has become much easier, raising the possibilities of success stories.

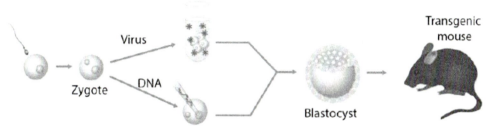

Figure: 30.2. Generation of gene-edited mouse by CRISPR/Cas9 by targeting the zygote (one-step process)

Cas9 RNA and guide RNA (gRNA) targeting a gene of interest is injected into the cytoplasm of the zygote. Mice carrying a mutation in both alleles of the targeted gene are derived in one step.

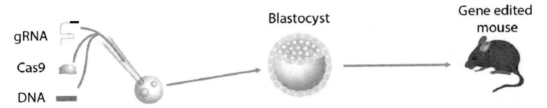

Figure: 30.3 Embryos at the 4 to 8 cell stage are infected with retroviruses or DNA is injected into the male pronucleus of the zygote.

The embryos can be transplanted into a foster mother. The exogenous DNA sequences are randomly integrated into the genome of the resulting transgenic mice directly or after incubation any time up until the blastocyst stage (~100 cells).

This technology has accelerated in vivo mouse model biomedical research. This mechanism has already been successfully used to target important genes in many cell lines and organisms. An exciting development is the use of the dCas9 version of the CRISPR/Cas9 system to target protein domains for transcriptional regulation (Perez Pinera, 2013), epigenetic modification (Hu, 2014), and microscopic visualization of specific genome loci (Chen et al, 2013). The proposed uses are on applying the technology to somatic cells (uncontroversial) but there is interest in using it to edit germline cells also. With germline cell and embryo genome editing (not legal in many countries) there are a number of ethical challenges, such as whether it can be allowed to enhance normal human traits thus tampering with the human genome in general, and not to remove disease which was the main purpose of these technologies being worked out. Nevertheless, the scenario is dynamic and ever-changing, research could propel the technology soon towards clinical use, with gene and cellular therapies put to efficient use for the cause of removing disease-causing genome sequences for improving the individual's quality of life.

Applications of CRISPR/Cas9 Technology:

1. Potential way to use CRISPR/Cas9 in cancer therapy could be the development of genetically engineered oncolytic viruses (Ovs).
2. Can be used in direct Cancer gene therapy.
3. Provides a new tool to manipulate non-coding regions of the cancer genes, accelerating the functional exploration of aspects that are not characterised yet.
4. To treat viral diseases. Provides a platform for antiviral therapeutics for treating infectious diseases, either by altering the host genes required by the virus or by targeting the viral genes necessary for replication.
5. To treat Allergy and immunological diseases.
6. CRISPR/Cas9 possesses potential against allergic and Mendelian disorders of the immune system.
7. Potential of CRISPR/Cas9 as antimicrobials.

Due to the robustness and flexibility of the technology, CRISPR has become a versatile tool with several other applications beyond genome-editing studies such as genome and chromatin manipulation efforts through catalytically impaired Cas9 enzymes, that are mainly repurposed to achieve targeted gene regulation, epigenome editing, chromatin imaging, and chromatin topology manipulations. The alternative application areas are mostly possible because of the programmable targeting capacity of catalytically inactive dead Cas9 (dCas9), which cannot cleave DNA but can still be guided to the target sequence (Figure 30.4).

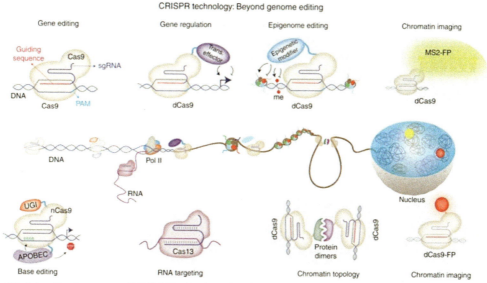

Figure: 30.4 Application areas of CRISPR-Cas based technologies beyond genome editing

During the pandemic that has currently gripped the world nations including India in 2020, India's first paper- strip test for Covid-19 used the cutting edge gene editing tool-Crispr/Cas9 to target and identifies the genomic sequences of the novel coronavirus in the samples of suspected individuals. This came as a boon in a situation when testing was of prime importance and we were short of testing kits for the same; until this innovation, a PCR based assay was used for testing the disease organism, most testing was initially done by NIV, Pune.

Given its promising performance, the gene editing technology has also promoted the development of cell imaging, gene expression regulation, epigenetic modification, therapeutic drug development, functional gene screening, and gene diagnosis. Although the off-target effect in the implementation of gene editing technology still needs further optimization, innovative genome editing complexes and more specific nanostructured vehicles have improved efficiency and reduced toxicity during the delivery process, bringing genome editing technology closer to the future therapeutics.

Glossary

Acrocentric: Chromosome with centromere near one end of short arm often with satellite.
Acentric: Chromosome without a centromere.
Allele: Alternative form of a gene.
Adenine: A purine base in DNA/ RNA.
Ancient DNA: Preserved DNA from an archaeological or fossil specimen.
Aneuploid: Chromosome number that is not an exact multiple of the haploid set, e.g. 2n-1 or 2n+1.
Anticodon: The complimentary triplet of tRNA molecule which binds to it with particular amino acid.
Antiparallel: Opposite orientation of 2 DNA strand one runs into 3' to 5' and the other 5' to 3' direction.
Archaeogenetics: The use of DNA analysis to study the human past.
Artificial gene synthesis: Construction of an artificial gene from a series of overlapping. oligonucleotides.
Autosomal dominant: A gene on the non sex chromosome which manifests in the heterozygous condition.
Autosomal inheritance: Pattern of inheritance shown by a disorder or trait determined by a gene of the non sex chromosome.
Autosomal recessive: A gene on the non sex chromosome which manifests in the heterozygous state.
Autosome: Any chromosome other than sex chromosome.
Base: Short for nitrogen base in nucleic acid A-adenine, T-thymine, U-Uracil C-cytosine, G-guanine.
B-DNA: Right handed double helical form of DNA of Watson and Crick.
Bioinformatics: The use of computer methods in studies of genomes.
Biotechnology: The use of biological processes in industry and technology.
Carrier: Healthy person possessing a mutant gene in heterozygous form.
C-DNA: Complimentary DNA, synthesized by reverse transcriptase.

Centimorgan: Chromosome mapping unit, one cM equals 1% recombinants in offsprings.
Central dogma: Concept that flow of genetic information is usually from DNA to RNA to protein.
Centromere: The point where 2 chromatids are joined, they control chromosome movement.
Chromatin: Nucleoprotein material of eukaryotic chromosome.
Chromatid: During cell division, each centromere divides longitudinally into 2 chromatids.
Chromosome: DNA complexed with RNA and histone protein forms a threadlike structure that contains genetic information in linear sequence.
Chromosome walking: A technique that can be used to construct a clone contig by identifying overlapping fragments of cloned DNA.
Chiasmata: X-shaped configuration formed at the point of contact between two chromatids belonging to homologous chromosomes.
Cistron: Smallest genetic unit of gene showing cis-trans function.
Cistrans: New terms for coupling and repulsion phase of linkage proposed by JBS Haldane.
Clone: Group of cells derived from a single cell, carry same genetic information.
Congenital: Any abnormality, genetic or not, present at birth.
Codominant: Trait resulting from expression of both alleles at a particular locus in heterozygotes, e.g. ABO blood groups.
Codon: Coding sequence of three adjacent nucleotides.
Codon bias: The fact that not all codons are used equally frequently in the genes of a particular organism.
Comparative genomics: A research strategy that uses information obtained from the study of one genome to make inferences about the map positions and functions of genes in a second genome.
CpG island: A GC-rich DNA region located upstream of approximately 56% of the genes in the human genome.
Cross over: Exchange of genetic material between homologous chromosomes during meiosis.
Cytogenetics: Branch of genetics which deals with transmission and behaviour of chromosomes.
Cytosine: A pyrimidine base in DNA and RNA.
Deletion: The loss of a part of a chromosome.
Diploid: Normal and Somatic cells containing 2 sets of 23 chromosomes.
DNA chip: A wafer of silicon carrying a high density array of oligonucleotides used in transcriptome and other studies.
DNA finger printing: Electrophoretic identification of individuals using DNA probes for highly polymorphic regions of the genome, such that the genome of every individual exhibits a unique pattern of bands.
DNA ladder: A mixture of DNA fragments, whose sizes are multiples of 100 bp or of 1 kb, used as size markers.
DNA marker: A DNA sequence that exists as two or more alleles and which can therefore be used in genetic mapping.

DNA polymerase: Enzyme that catalyses synthesis of DNA from deoxynucleoside 5' triphosphates under the direction of a DNA template strand

DNA sequencing: Determination of the order of nucleotides in a DNA molecule

Dominant: An allele expressed in heterozygous

Duplication: A chromosome is larger than normal, the extra segment being identical to a segment of the normal chromosome

Dysmorphology: Study of malformations arising from abnormal embryogenesis

Empirical risk: Risk of recurrence for multifactorial/polygenic disorders based on family studies

Euchromatin: Genetic material that is not stained so intensely by certain dyes during interphase

Euploid: A complete set of chromosomes, the total number being 92, incompatible with life

Exon: Sequence of gene retained in mRNA after the intrans are removed from the primary transcript

Fluorescence in situ **hybridization (FISH):** A hybridization technique that uses fluorochromes of different colors to enable two or more genes to be located within a chromosome preparation in a single *in situ* experiment

Forward genetics: The strategy by which the genes responsible for a phenotype are identified by determining which genes are inactivated in organisms that display a mutant version of that phenotype

Fragile site: A chromosome segment that has a tendency to break

Fragile X-syndrome: Syndrome involving X chromosome associated with mental retardation, X chromosome tip breaks

Functional genomics: Studies aimed at identifying all the genes in a genome and determining their expression patterns and functions

G-bands: Giemsa bands (stained with Giemsa stain) in eukaryotic chromosome

Gene: Unit of inheritance (DNA) is a fixed position on a chromosome determines a specific biologic function

Gene therapy: A clinical procedure in which a gene or other DNA sequence is used to treat/manage a disease

Genetics: The science of heredity and variation

Genetic code: The linear sequences of nucleotides that specify the amino acids during translation at ribosome

Genetic counselling: Process by which information on genetic disorders is given to the family

Genotype: Genes that an organism possesses, genetic constitution

Genetic engineering: The use of experimental techniques to produce DNA molecules containing new genes or new combinations of genes

Genetic fingerprinting: A hybridization technique that determines the genomic distribution of a hyper variable dispersed repetitive sequence and results in a banding pattern that is specific for each individual

Genetic map: A genome map that has been obtained by analysing the results of genetic crosses

Genome: A complete set of haploid (23) chromosomes (hence of genes) inherited as a unit from one

parent.
Genomics: The study of a genome, in particular the complete sequencing of a genome
Genomic library: Set of cloned fragments making up the entire genome of an organism
Guanine: A purine base in DNA/RNA
Haploid: Normal gametes containing haploid (n=23) chromosome
Hemizygote: Male genotype with X-linked trait, as male have XY it is called hemizygote
Heterozygote: Person possessing different alleles at a particular locus on homologous chromosome
Holandric inheritance: Pattern of inheritance of genes on the Y chromosome inheritance
Homologous chromosome: Chromosome that pair at meiosis at a particular locus homologous chromosome
Homologous recombination: Recombination between two homologous double-stranded DNA molecules, i.e., ones which share extensive nucleotide sequence similarity
Homozygote: Person having two identical alleles at a particular locus on homologous chromosome
HGP: Human genome project
Heritability: The contribution of genetic as opposed to environmental factors to phenotype variance
In situ hybridisation: A technique for gene mapping involving hybridization of a labeled sample of a cloned gene to a large DNA molecule, usually a chromosome
In vitro mutagenesis: Any one of several techniques used to produce a specified mutation at a predetermined position in a DNA molecule
Ionizing radiations: Electromagnetic waves (X and g rays) and high energy particles (neutrons)
Jumping genes: Transposable elements (TEs) DNA sequences that move from one location on the genome to another
Karyotype: Descriptions of chromosomes based on various characters
Kilobase (Kb): 1000 base pairs of DNA
Ligase (DNA ligase): An enzyme that, in the cell, repairs single-stranded discontinuities in double-stranded DNA molecules. Purified DNA ligase is used in gene cloning to join DNA molecules together
Linkage: Association of loci on the same chromosome they are inherited together hence, linked
Linkage analysis: A technique for mapping the chromosomal position of a gene by comparing its inheritance pattern with that of genes and other loci whose map positions are already known
Linkage map: A linear diagram that shows the relative positions of genes on a chromosome a determined by genetic analysis
Locus (plural- loci): The position of a gene on a chromosome
Lyonisation: Process of one of the X-chromosome inactivation in every cell of a female during early embryonic development
Marker: A locus/allele whose phenotype provides information about a chromosome/segment during genetic analysis.
Mass spectrometry: An analytical technique in which ions are separated according to their mass-to-charge ratios

Matrix-assisted laser desorption ionization time-of-flight (MALDI-TOF): A type of mass spectrometry used in proteomics.
Meiosis: Cell division during gametogenesis resulting in haploid gametes.
Messenger RNA (mRNA): The transcript of a protein-coding gene.
Metacentric: A chromosome whose centromere is in the middle.
Microarray: A set of genes or cDNAs immobilized on a glass slide and used in transcriptome studies.
Mitochondrial DNA: The DNA molecules present in the mitochondria of eukaryotes.
Mitochondrial Eve: The woman who lived in Africa between 140,000 and 290,000 years ago and who carried the ancestral mitochondrial DNA that gave rise to all the mitochondrial DNAs in existence today.
Mitosis: Cell division in somatic cells.
Monosomy: Loss of one of a pair of homologous chromosomes.
Mosaic: Presence of two different cell lines derived from a single zygote.
Multifactorial inheritance: A trait determined by the combined action of many factors, typically some genetic and some environmental.
Multiple alleles: Occurrence in a population of more than two alleles of a gene.
Mutation: Sudden heritable change in chromosome or DNA.
Mutagen: An agent capable of causing mutation/enhancing mutation rate.
Muton: Smallest mutable site within a cistron.
Non-disjunction: Failure of separation of paired chromosomes during meiosis.
Northern blotting: A gel transfer technique used for RNA.
Nucleoside: A sugar base compound that is nucleotide precursor.
Nucleotide: consist of a nitrogen base, a sugar and one or more phosphate group.
Oncogene: gene with the potential to cause cancer.
Oncogenetics: Genetic study of cancer.
Out of Africa hypothesis: A hypothesis that holds that modern humans evolved in Africa, moving to the rest of the Old World between 100 000 and 50 000 years ago, displacing the descendants of *Homo erectus* that they encountered.
Pedigree analysis: The use of a human family tree to analyze the inheritance of a genetic or DNA marker.
Penetrance: Probability that a disease genotype will result in an abnormal phenotype.
Pharming: Genetic modification of a farm animal so that the animal synthesizes a recombinant pharmaceutical protein, often in its milk.
Phenotype: Physical characteristics of a person reflecting genetic constitution and environmental influence.
Physical map: A genome map that has been obtained by direct examination of DNA molecules.
Peptide mass fingerprinting: Identification of a protein by examination of the mass spectrometer.
Polygenic inheritance: Disorder/trait caused by interaction between many genes.

Polymerase chain reaction (PCR): A method to amplify rapid by DNA segments in cycles of denaturation, primer addition and replication.

Polymorphism: Refers to a locus that is present as a number of different alleles or other variations in the population as a whole.

Polyploid: Chromosome numbers representing multiples of the haploid set greater than diploid e.g. 3n, 4n, etc.

Post-genomics: Studies aimed at identifying all the genes in a genome and determining their expression patterns and functions.

Proband: The person through whom a pedigree is discovered.

Probe: a radioactive DNA/RNA molecule used in DNA/ RNA hybridisation assays.

Proteome: The entire protein content of a cell or tissue.

Proteomics: The collection of techniques used to study the proteome.

Pseudogene: Functionless copy of a known gene.

Recessive: An allele that does not express itself in heterozygous condition .

Recombination: Crossing over between homologous chromosomes at meiosis which separates linked loci.

Recombinant: A transformed cell that contains a recombinant DNA molecule.

Recombinant DNA molecule: A DNA molecule created in the test tube by ligating together pieces of DNA that are not normally contiguous.

Recombinant DNA technology: All of the techniques involved in the construction, study and use of recombinant DNA molecules.

Recon: Smallest recombinanatle unit within a cistron.

Restriction endonuclease: Enzyme that recognizes certain DNA sequences which they cleave.

Restriction digest: Result of action of restriction endonuclease on DNA sample.

Restriction maps: A physical map of a piece of DNA showing recognition sites of specific restriction endonuclease separated by lengths marked in number of bases.

Restriction fragment length polymorphism (RFLP): Variations in banding patterns of electrophoresed restriction digest.

Reverse genetics: The strategy by which the function of a gene is identified by mutating that gene and identifying the phenotypic change that results.

Reverse transcriptase: An RNA-dependent DNA polymerase, able to synthesize a complementary.

Ribonuclease: An enzyme that degrades RNA.

Segregation: Separation of alleles during meiosis so that each gamete contains only one member of each pair of alleles.

Serial analysis of gene expression (SAGE): A method for studying the composition of a transcriptome.

Sex chromosome: Chromosome other than autosome that determine sex of the organism.

Sex linked: Inheritance pattern of genes located on sex chromosome, X-linked or Y-linkage.

Southern blotting: Method used to transfer DNA fragments from an agarose gel to a mitrocellulose gel for the purpose of DNA-DNA or DNA-RNA hybridisation during r-DNA work.

Sub-metacentric: A chromosome whose centromere is away from the centre of chromosome.

Synapsis: Point by point pairing of homologous chromosome during zygotene of meiosis.

Synteny: Refers to a pair of genomes in which at least some of the genes are located at similar map positions.

Thermal cycle sequencing: A DNA sequencing method that uses PCR to generate chain terminated polynucleotides.

Transcription: Process by which the information contained in the coding strand of DNA is copied into a single stranded RNA molecule of complementary base sequence.

Trait: Recognizable pheonotype due to a genetic character.

Translation: Process of protein synthesis where in the primary structure of the protein is determined by the nucleotide sequence in mRNA.

Translocation: A portion of a chromosome attached to another chromosome.

Triploid: Cells containing three haploids sets of chromosomes (3n).

Triplet code: A series of 3 bases in DNA/RNA molecule which codes for a specific amino acid.

Terminator codons (Stop codons): UAC – also called Amber codon, UAA – also called Ochre codon.

Thymine: A pyrimidine base in DNA.

Trisomy: Cells containing one more than the normal diploid set of chromosome (2n+1).

Unifactorial: Inheritance controlled by a single gene pair.

Uracil: A pyrimidine base in RNA.

Vector: A plasmid into which foreign DNA can be inserted for cloning.

Watson–Crick rules: The base pairing rules that underlie gene structure and expression. A pairs with T, and G pairs with C.

Western Blotting: Technique for probing for a particular protein using antibodies.

YAC: Yeast artificial chromosome capable of cloning very large pieces of DNA useful in Human Genome Research work.

Y-linked: Inheritance pattern of genes on Y chromosome (also called holandric genes).

Z-DNA: Left handed double helical DNA.

Bibliography

1. Abbas AR, Baldwin D, Ma Y, Ouyang W, Gurney A, Martin F, Fong S, van Lookeren Campagne M, Godowski P, Williams PM, Chan AC, Clark HF. Immune response in silico (IRIS): immune-specific genes identified from a compendium of microarray expression data. Genes Immun. 2005 Jun; 6(4):319-31.
2. Ahuja, Yog & Sharma, Sanjeev & Bahadur, Bir. (2013). Autism: An epigenomic side-effect of excessive exposure to electromagnetic fields. Int J of Medicine and Medical Sci 5. 171-177.
3. Anderson, W.F. **1992**. Human gene therapy. *Science*, **256** : 808-813.
4. Bianchi E, Doe B, Goulding D, Wright GJ. Juno is the egg Izumo receptor and is essential for mammalian fertilization. Nature. 2014;508:483–487.
5. Sahijram, Leela & Maligeppagol, Manamohan, Kanupriya, Rao, B., Bahadur, Bir. (2016). Methylomics and inheritance in plants: DNA and RNA methylation. Genetics and Molecular Biology in Crop Improvement, Chapter: 6, Publisher: Pointer Publishers, Jaipur, Editors: P.C. Trivedi, pp.130-171.
6. Budowle B, Connell ND, Bielecka-Oder A, Colwell RR, Corbett CR, Fletcher J, et al. Validation of high throughput sequencing and microbial forensics applications. Investig Genet. 2014;5:9. pmid:25101166; PubMed Central PMCID: PMCPMC4123828.
7. Bridges C. B., Morgan T. H. (1923). The Third-Chromosome Group of Mutant Characters of Drosophila melanogaster (Carnegie Institution of Washington publication, no. 327), pp. 1–251. Washington, DC: Carnegie Institution of Washington.
8. Carrington M, Walker BD. Immunogenetics of spontaneous control of HIV. Annu Rev Med. 2012; 63:131-45.
9. Casperson, T. Farber, S. and Foley, G. E. **1968**. Chemical differentiation along metaphase chromosome *Exp cell Res.* **42** : 219.
10. Cavence, W. L. and R.L. White. **1995**. Genetic basis of cancer. Sci. Amer, **272** : 72-79.
11. Chen, B., et al. (2013) *Cell*, 155, 1479–1491.

12. Clarke, A. **1992.** *Genetic counselling.* Routledge, London.
13. Coleman, G. C. and Nelson J. F. *Principles of Oral diagnosis,* Mosby, N.J., U.S.A.
14. Cummings, M.R. **1991.** *Human heredity.* West, St Paul., U.S.A.
15. Derlica, K. **1984.** *Understanding gene cloning.* Wiley, USA.
16. Derouchy, J. and Turlean, C. **1984** *Clinical atlas of human chromosomes.* Wiley, New York, USA
17. Donis, Keller, H. **1990.** *Human genome mapping techniques* Stockton Press, New York.
18. Donnai, D, Winter, R.M. **1995.** *Congenital malformations syndromes.* Chapman and Hall London.
19. Driscoll, D.A., Spinner, N. B., Budarf, M. L. **1992.** Deletions and microdeletions of 22q 11/2 in velo-cardio-facial syndrome. *Amer. J.Med. Genet,* **44** : 261.
20. Dunn, L.C. **1965.** *A short history of genetics.* McGraw Hill, USA.
21. Farrow, M. and Juberg, R. **1969.** Genetics and law prohibiting marriages in the United Sates. *J. Amer. Med. Assoc,* **209** : 534-538.
22. Friedman, J. M., Dill, F. J., Hayden, M. R. and McGillivary, B.C. **1997.** *Genetics.* N.M.S. series, Waverly, N. Delhi (reprint).
23. Garber, E.O. **1972.** *Cytogenetics.* McGraw Hill, USA.
24. Garrod, A.E. **1909.** *Inborn errors of metabolism.* Hodder and Stoughton, London.
25. Gorlin, R.J., Cohen, M.M., Levine, L.S. **1990.** *Syndromes of the head and neck.* 3rd edn. Oxford University Press, Oxford.
26. Gray, J.W. et. al. **1987.** *High speed chromosome sorting.* Science. **238** : 323-329.
27. Hamblin TJ, Davis Z, Gardiner A, Oscier DG, Stevenson FK. Unmutated Ig V(H) genes are associated with a more aggressive form of chronic lymphocytic leukemia. Blood. 1999;94(6): 1848–54.
28. Harth, Daniel, L. **1991.** *Basic genetics.* Jones and Bartlett, Boston, USA.
29. Horner DS, Pavesi G, Castrignano T, De Meo PD, Liuni S, Sammeth M, et al. Bioinformatics approaches for genomics and post genomics applications of next-generation sequencing. Brief Bioinform. 2010;11(2):181–97. pmid:19864250.
30. Huu, J., et al. (2014) *Nucleic Acids Res.* doi:10.1093/nar/gku109.
31. Innes, M.A., Gelfaud, D.H., Snicsky and White, T.J. **1989.***PCR protocols : A guide to methodologies and applications.* Academic Press, San Diego, USA.
32. Kingston, H.M. **1997.** *ABC of Clinical Genetics.* BMJ Publisher. Kent. UK.
33. Kirby, L.T. **1990.** *DNA finger printing : An introduction.* Stockton Press, New York.
34. Kumar, B., Shetty, V. and Valiathan, A. **1998.** Incidence of cleft lip and palate in Manipal in the fast decade. *Indian J. Orofacial Genetics.* **1** : 16-19.
35. Lan JH, Zhang Q. Clinical applications of next-generation sequencing in histocompatibility and transplantation. Curr Opin Organ Transplant. 2015 Aug;20(4):461-7.
36. Lejeune, J, Gauthier M, Turpin R. **1959.** Etude des chromosomes somatiques de neuf enfants mongoliens. *CR. Acad. Sci.* (Paris) : **248** : 1721-1722.
37. Lewis R **1994** : *Human geneticsConcepts and applications.* W.C. Brown Iowa, USA.

38. Madhavi M, Vinukonda S, Prasannalatha K, Nagula P, Rekha rani K, Premsagar K, Sagurthi S.R.(2019). Association of *CDKN2BAS* gene polymorphism with periodontitis and Coronary Artery Disease from South Indian population. Gene, Vol 710:324-332.
39. Magalini, S. I., Magalini S. C., de Francisci G. **1990**. *Dictionary of medical syndromes*, ed 3, Philadelphia, Lippincott.
40. Mamta B, Bahadur, Bir, MV, Rajam. (2016). RNA silencing: A novel tool for crop protection against Biotic and abiotic stresses.. In; Plant Stress Physiology. Ed.Trivedi PC. Special VolumePointer Publishers, Jaipur India,ISBN 978-81-7132-832-1. 147-163.
41. Mark, H.F.L., Hanna, I. And Gnepp D. R. **1996**. Cytogenetic analysis of salivary gland tumours. *Oral Surg. Oral Med. Oral Pathol. Oral Radiol. Endod* **82**:187
42. McKubick, V.A. **1994**. *Mendelian inheritance in man*. 11th edn. 2 vols. John Hopkins., Univ. Press Baltimore.
43. McKusick, V.A. **1971**. The mapping of human chromosome. *Sci. Amer.* (April).
44. McKusick, V.A. **1998**. The new genetics and clinical medicine. *Hospit. Pract.* 23 : 177-191.
45. Meyers, R. A. (ed). **1996**. *Encyclopedia of Molecular Biology and Molecular Medicine* VCH Verlagsgesellschaft. Federal Republic of Germany.
46. Milterlman, F., Johansson, B., Mandahl, N. **1997**. Clinical significance of cytogeentic findings in solid tumours. *Cancer Gentic Cytogenet*. **95**:1.
47. Muliken, J. B., Warman, M. L. **1996**. Molecular genetic and craniofacial surgery. *Plast Reconstruction Surg*. **97** : 666.
48. Muller, H.J. **1927**. Artificial transmutation of gene. *Science*., 66 : 84-87.
49. Mulligan, R.C. **1993**. Gene therapy. Science. 260 : 926-936.
50. Nederlof PM, Robinson D, Abuknesha R, Wiegant J, Hopman AH, Tanke HJ, Raap AK: Threecolor fluorescence in situ hybridization for the simultaneous detection of multiple nucleic acid sequences. Cytometry 10:20-27, 1989.
51. Palca, J. **1990**. The other human genome. Science. 249 : 1104-1105.
52. Perez-Pinera, P., et al. (2013) *Nat. Methods,* 10, 239–242.
53. Peters, J.A. **1959**. Classical papers in genetics. Prentice Hall, New Jersey.
54. Poole, Andrew E **1975**. Dental clinics of North America (Symposium on Genetics). Vol 19 (1) : 1-210.
55. Prabhu, S. R., Wilson, D. F., Daftary, D. K., Johnson, N. W. **1993**. Oral diseases in the tropics, Oxford University Press, Bombay.
56. *Primakoff P, Myles DG*. Penetration, adhesion, and fusion in mammalian sperm-egg interaction. *Science. 2002 Jun 21; 296(5576):2183-5.*
57. Reed EF. Technical and conceptual advances in histocompatibility and immunogenetics inform on mechanisms of transplant rejection and pave the way to development of novel therapies. Curr Opin Organ Transplant. 2015 Aug;20(4):444-5.

58. Reddy, R. N. **1983**. Cleft lip and palate: A study on epidemiology and genetics. Masters degree dissertation, Mangalore University.
59. Regezi, J. A. and Seiubba J. J. Oral pathology, W. B. Saunders Co. London.
60. Risch, N **1992**. Genetics linkage, interpreting lod scores. Science, 255-803-804.
61. Robert, F., Mueller and Ian D Young **1998**. Emerys elements of medical genetics. Churchill Livingston, Edinburgh.
62. Sambrook, J., E. F. Fritsch and T. Maniatis **1989**. Molecular Cloning: A laboratory Manual. Cold Spring Harbour Lab. Press. New York.
63. Schauman, B **1976**. Dermatoglyphics in Medical disorders Springer Verlag, Berlin.
64. Schaumann, B. and M. Alter 1994. Dermatoglyphics in Medical Disorders, Springer Verlag, N.Y.
65. Schuettengruber B., Chourrout D., Vervoort M., Leblanc B., Cavalli G. (2007). Genome regulation by polycomb and trithorax proteins. Cell 128, 735–745.
66. Singson A, Zannoni S, Kadandale P. Molecules that function in the steps of fertilization. Cytokine Growth Factor Rev. 2001 Dec; 12(4):299-304.
67. Snustad, D. P., Simmons, M. J. Jenkins, J. B. **1997**. Principles of Genetics. Wiley. New York.
68. Srb, A, Owen, R. R. Edgar. **1975**. General Genetics, Freeman U.S.A.
69. Stephens, J.C., M. L. Cavanangle and M. L. Gradie, M. L. Mador and K. L. Kidd. **1990**. Mapping the human genome: Current status. Science., 250:237.
70. Stern, C. **1973**. Principles of Human Genetics. W. H. Freeman, San Francisco.
71. Sturtevant, A. H. **1965**. A History of Genetics, Harper and Row New York.
72. Summer, A. T. **1990**. *Chromosome Banding*. Unwin Hyman, Cambridge, Mass.
73. Swanson, C. P. **1957**. *Cytology and Cytogenetics*. Prentice Hall, New York.
74. Sykes, B. **1985**. Molecular genetics of collagen. *Bio Essays*, 3:112-117.
75. Tamarin, R. H. **1993**. *Principles of Genetics*. W. C. Brown, Iowa, U.S.A.
76. Tantawy AAG. Immunogenetics of type 1 diabetes mellitus Egypt J Pediatr Allergy Immunol 2008; 6(1): 3-12.
77. Therman, Eeva and M. Susman **1993**. *Human Chromosome-Structure, Behaviour and effects*. Springer Verlag, New York Berlin.
78. Thompson, M. W., P. R. McInnes and H. F. Willard **1991**. *Genetics in Medicine*. Saunders, Philadelphia.
79. Tijo, J. H. and Levan, A. **1956**. The Chromosome number of man. *Hereditas*. 42:1-6.
80. Todd, R, Donoff, R. B. and Wong D. T. W. **2000**. The chromosome : cytogenetic analysis and its clinical applications. *J. Oral Maxillofac. Surg.* 58 : 1034 – 1039.
81. Valentine, G. **1975**. *Chromosome disorders. An introduction for clinicians*. Lippincott. Philadelphia U.S.A.
82. Vasavi, M. Ahuja, Y.R. & Hasan, Q. **2012**. Muscular myopathies other than myotonic dystrophy also associated with (CTG)n expansion at the DMPK locus. Journal of pediatric neurosciences. 7. 175-178.

83. M Vasavi, S Ponnala, K Gujjari, P Boddu, RS Bharatula, R Prasad et al. (2005). DNA methylation in esophageal diseases including cancer: special reference to hMLH1 gene promoter methylation status. Tumori Journal 92 (2), 155-162.
84. Verma, R. and A. Babu **1989**. *Human Chromosome. Manual of Basic techniques.* Pergamon Press. New York.
85. Verna, I. M. **1990**. Gene Therapy. *Sci.Amer.*
86. Vogel, F. **1992**. Risk Calculations for Hereditary effects of ionising radiations in Man. *Human Genet*, **89**:127-146.
87. Wallace, D.C. **1989**. Mitochondrial mutations and neuromuscular diseases. *Trends in Genet*, 5:9.
88. Watson, J. D. **1968**. *The Double Helix.* Signet, New York, U.S.A.
89. White, R **1992**. Inherited Cancer Genes. *Curr. Opin, Genet. Dev.*, **2**:53-57.
90. Younis, I. **1983**. The chromosomal basis and human neoplasia. *Science*, **221** : 227-2.